The Inflammatory Bowel Disease Yearbook 2004

Remedica State of the Art series
ISSN 1472-4626

Also available
The Handbook of Diabetes Mellitus and Cardiovascular Disease
Kidney Transplantation
The Inflammatory Bowel Disease Yearbook 2003
Management of Atherosclerotic Carotid Disease
Multiple Myeloma
Rheumatoid Arthritis
Viral Co-infections in HIV: Impact and Management

Published by Remedica
32–38 Osnaburgh Street, London, NW1 3ND, UK
Civic Opera Building, 20 North Wacker Drive, Suite 1642, Chicago, IL 60606, USA

Email: info@remedicabooks.com
www.remedicabooks.com

Publisher: Andrew Ward
In-house editor: Cath Harris
Design: AS&K Skylight Creative Services

While every effort is made by the publisher to see that no inaccurate or misleading
data, opinions, or statements appear in this book, they wish to make it clear that
the material contained in the publication represents a summary of the independent
evaluations and opinions of the editor and contributors. As a consequence, the
editor, authors, publisher, and any sponsoring company accept no responsibility
for the consequences of any inaccurate or misleading data or statements. Neither
do they endorse the content of the publication or the use of any drug or device
in a way that lies outside its current licensed application in any territory.

Remedica is a member of the AS&K Media Partnership.

ISBN 1 901346 81 1
British Library Cataloguing-in-Publication Data
A catalogue record for this book is available from the British Library.

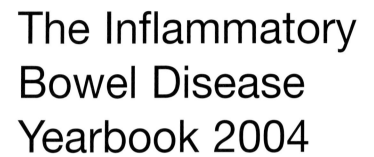

The Inflammatory Bowel Disease Yearbook 2004

Charles N Bernstein, MD, Editor

Professor of Medicine
Head, Section of Gastroenterology
Director, Inflammatory Bowel Disease Clinical and Research Centre
University of Manitoba
Winnipeg, Manitoba, Canada

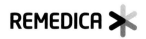

Authors

Ian DR Arnott, MD
Gastrointestinal Unit
University of Edinburgh Department of Medical Sciences
School of Clinical and Molecular Medicine
Western General Hospital
Edinburgh, UK

Charles N Bernstein, MD
Professor of Medicine
Head, Section of Gastroenterology
Director, Inflammatory Bowel Disease Clinical and
Research Centre
University of Manitoba
Winnipeg, Manitoba, Canada

Kenneth Croitoru, MDCM, FRCP(C)
Professor of Medicine, Intestinal Disease Research Program
Division of Gastroenterology
McMaster University
Hamilton, Ontario, Canada

Donald R Duerksen, MD, FRCP(C)
Associate Professor of Medicine
St Boniface General Hospital and University of Manitoba
Director, Manitoba Home Nutrition Program
Winnipeg, Manitoba, Canada

Steven H Itzkowitz, MD
The Dr Burrill B Crohn Professor of Medicine
Associate Director, The Dr Henry D Janowitz Division
of Gastroenterology
Department of Medicine
The Mount Sinai School of Medicine
New York, USA

Robin S McLeod, MD
Professor of Surgery and Health Policy, Management
and Evaluation
University of Toronto
Head, Division of General Surgery
Mount Sinai Hospital
Toronto, Ontario, Canada

Jack Satsangi, DPhil, FRCP
Professor of Gastroenterology
Gastrointestinal Unit
University of Edinburgh Department of Medical Sciences
School of Clinical and Molecular Medicine
Western General Hospital
Edinburgh, UK

Preface

The Inflammatory Bowel Disease Yearbook 2004 is the second edition of our annual IBD update. With each yearbook, our goal is to present six state of the art reviews for IBD investigators and clinicians. This is a review of the latest data pertinent to each topic – to ensure it is up-to-date, our yearbook is written and published within the same calendar year.

This year, we have brought together another outstanding group of highly regarded authors. Ken Croitoru of McMaster University reviews current concepts regarding the pathogenesis of IBD. With the discovery of the *CARD15* gene mutations in Crohn's disease and with a heightened interest in the potential of either exogenous or endogenous (bowel flora) microbes in triggering the inflammatory response, more comprehensive pathogenetic paradigms are emerging.

Ian Arnott and Jack Satsangi of the University of Edinburgh provide an update on IBD classifications, reviewing genetic and serologic markers as well as phenotyping paradigms. Subtyping IBD has emerged as an important aspect of dissecting disease pathogenesis, and markers that facilitate stricter subtyping are being avidly pursued. Don Duerksen of the University of Manitoba then reviews nutritional deficiencies and nutritional therapies in IBD, including the use of total parenteral nutrition, percutaneous gastrostomy feeding tubes, and specialized diets.

Robin McLeod from the University of Toronto addresses the current approaches to surgery in IBD. Her chapter reviews issues related to surgery in Crohn's disease, ileoanal pouch procedures for ulcerative colitis, and laparoscopic approaches in both diseases. This year's edition also provides updates on two important complications of IBD. Steven Itzkowitz from the Mount Sinai School of Medicine reviews colorectal cancer in IBD, including issues related to low-grade dysplasia, a diagnosis that still engenders debate about clinical management. Finally, I provide a review of osteoporosis in IBD and present a view on pursuing bone density testing in IBD. Bone density testing has become overused in IBD as emerging fracture data have been discordant with the plethora of bone density data that suggest a high rate of osteoporosis.

You will find *The Inflammatory Bowel Disease Yearbook 2004* to be a thorough update of these important topical issues in IBD, and we look forward to presenting a new yearbook in 2005.

Charles N Bernstein, MD
University of Manitoba Inflammatory Bowel Disease
Clinical and Research Centre
Winnipeg, Manitoba, Canada

Contents

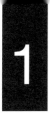

Pathogenesis

Kenneth Croitoru

Introduction

The current model of the pathogenesis of inflammatory bowel disease (IBD) attempts to understand the obvious chronic inflammatory process in the context of observations regarding genetic predisposition, a recently identified genetic mutation, and observational and case-control studies that suggest a possible influence of environmental factors. Simply put, the resulting paradigm is that IBD results from a dysregulated immune response to environmental trigger(s) in a genetically susceptible host. Advances in our understanding of the contributions of each of these elements and their interactions in defining the IBD patient are a result of studies in both animal models of the disease and in humans. Progress in these arenas has led to significant breakthroughs that are also relevant to other chronic inflammatory diseases. This chapter reviews selected areas in which advances have been made.

Lessons from case-control and natural history studies of patients

The analysis of large case-control studies continues to highlight potential clues regarding the etiology and pathogenesis of IBD, and focuses our attention on possible environmental factors or events that remain to be defined in individual patients or even in experimental animal models. The classic example is the observation that smoking is negatively associated with ulcerative colitis (UC), but associated with a worsening of Crohn's disease (CD) [1,2]. These observations have yet to be explained mechanistically. Unfortunately, attempts to take advantage of this observation by using nicotine in the treatment of UC patients have not been very successful [3,4].

In an important series of studies that analyzed large databases for cohort behavior, Sonnenberg and colleagues highlighted an intriguing observation regarding a cohort effect in terms of IBD epidemiologic trends, suggesting an environmental exposure that is diminishing with time [5–7]. A further observation was of a negative association between a history of appendectomy and UC [8,9]. A similar observation has been made in an animal model of colitis (using T-cell receptor [TCR]α knockout mice), raising the possibility that the underlying mechanism of such a relationship could be defined [10].

Lessons from human genetic studies

The identification of *NOD2/CARD15* mutations as the basis for the *IBD1* gene locus association with CD represents one of the most significant breakthroughs in human genetic studies of complex multigenic diseases [11–13]. The relevance of a mutation in a gene thought to represent an intracellular receptor of bacterial peptidoglycans suggests an important relationship of CD with enteric bacteria, but this remains to be defined [14–16]. The clinical phenotype of patients in the context of their *NOD2* allelotype has been explored [17–21], with results suggesting that this mutation may influence disease expression.

The exact role of the *NOD2* gene in the pathogenesis of IBD continues to be the focus of investigation. It would appear that NOD2 can function as a bacterial sensor through its ability to interact with bacterial components. Whether this confers a protective role against bacterial pathogens is not known. Indeed, the *NOD2* gene is expressed on intestinal epithelial cells and Paneth cells, which produce elements of innate immunity (eg, defensins) [22–24]. It remains to be determined how a defect in this pathway would lead to increased intestinal inflammation – although mice with a defect in nuclear factor-κB, one of the targets of *NOD2* activation, develop intestinal inflammation [25].

While the focus on bacteria may be appropriate, it is worth noting that the *NOD2* gene is also involved in apoptotic pathways, although the mutations defined for CD patients have not mapped to this region of the gene [14]. As other disease-associated genetic loci are identified, the challenge will be to understand the functional relevance of these genes in terms of pathogenesis [26].

Lessons from animal models

Since the initial identification of spontaneous colitis in mice with targeted mutations of genes involved in immune function (eg, interleukin [IL]-2, IL-10, and TCRα knockout mice [27–29]), there are now over 30 animal models of intestinal inflammation [30–32]. These models are based on defined genetic mutations or a variety of immune manipulations. Most of these models focus on the mucosal–environment interface as the site of interaction between host and intestinal microbes or bacterial flora. Indeed, the most consistent observation in these models is their dependence on gut flora for the expression of intestinal inflammation. These models therefore recapitulate the thesis that IBD results from an inappropriate immune response to an environmental factor, possibly a microbe, in a genetically susceptible host (see **Figure 1**). Therefore, the areas of investigation aim to define defects in barrier function, immune responses, and immune regulation, and altered enteric flora constituents. Defined genetic defects may be central to these events and influence their expression.

Defects in epithelial barrier function

Human studies have suggested that IBD patients have intestinal epithelial permeability defects that may precede the onset of

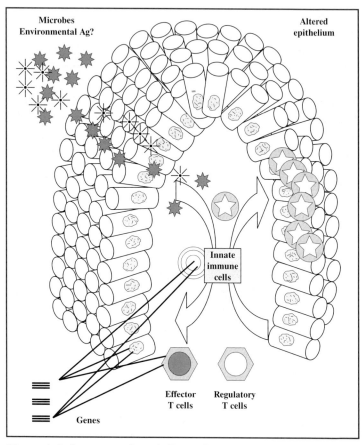

Figure 1. Inflammatory bowel disease is the result of the interaction between the local immune response and the enteric flora. This schematic diagram depicts the genetic influence on the interaction between the host immune system and environmental antigens or microbes.

clinical inflammation [33], which indicates the expression of a genetically determined predisposition [34]. Animal models that illustrate how altered barrier function may lead to or contribute to intestinal inflammation include those with genetically modified *N*-cadherin, a protein involved in homotypic cell interactions in the intestinal epithelium [35]. Defects in trefoil factor, a peptide that confers a degree of epithelial integrity in response to injury, have also been shown to lead to intestinal inflammation [36]. In addition, peptides with trophic activity on the intestinal epithelium have been studied in the context of improving inflammation [37,38].

More recently, mice defective in the multidrug resistance gene (*mdr1a–/–*) have been shown to develop spontaneous colitis [39]. Bone marrow transfer studies suggest that this genetic mutation is expressed via the nonhematologic cellular elements of the intestine. How this relates to altered barrier function and altered exposure to enteric flora remains to be defined, but, in a series of intriguing studies, the authors showed that *Helicobacter* species influenced the development of colitis in *mdr-1* knockout mice, with *H.bilis* infection accelerating and *H.hepaticus* infection delaying the development of colitis [40]. Therefore, the role of the "barrier" in the development of IBD is clearly important, although it remains to be defined.

Defects in immune function

Despite the great strides that have been taken in developing animal models with specific defects in immune function that lead to the development of intestinal inflammation, human studies have failed to define a consistent abnormality in immune function in either CD or UC patients. Nonetheless, definition of the cellular and molecular elements involved in the immune response in animal models of normal and inflamed intestine continues to provide exciting advances in therapeutic target development, and has contributed to the increasing numbers of biological therapies that are being evaluated in clinical trials. Therefore, defining normal and abnormal immune mechanisms in animal models continues to be fruitful as we struggle to define the human equivalent of these immune abnormalities in patients with IBD.

Altered B-cell function
Human studies have tried to define an autoimmune mechanism to IBD and have searched for pathogenic autoantibodies in

affected patients. A number of autoantibodies with potential pathogenetic relevance have been identified, although there is uncertainty as to their exact role in disease initiation and perpetuation. Two such autoantibodies, perinuclear antineutrophil cytoplasmic antibody (pANCA) and anti-*Saccharomyces cerevisiae* antibody (ASCA), are of some clinical value in identifying patients with IBD and aid in discriminating between CD and UC [41–43].

More recent studies have defined two autoantibodies in CD patients, OmpC and I2 [44–46]. These probably recognize bacterial determinants, implying a loss of normal tolerance to bacterial antigen. These findings suggest that enteric bacteria are stimulating the immune system and leading to the development of these antibodies. It remains to be determined whether the expression of these autoantibodies represents an intrinsic defect in B-cell function, a loss of T-cell regulation, or simply a response to an antigen that is not normally exposed to the local immune system. It is worth noting that a role has been defined for B cells with regulatory function in studies of TCRα knockout mice [47]. This observation needs to be explored further in both animal models and humans.

Altered T-cell function

Technological advances in cellular and molecular immunology have improved our ability to study T-cell function *in vitro* and *in vivo*. Nonetheless, it remains difficult to define specific T-cell abnormalities in a complex inflammatory disease (such as IBD) in the absence of a known antigenic target (ie, defining the T-cell specificity, as has been done for celiac disease). Nonetheless, it remains plausible that no specific antigen drives T-cell responses in patients with IBD, but rather an abnormality in the regulatory function serves to globally control inappropriate immune responses, which, in the context of IBD, revolve around responses to the normal gut flora.

New developments in our understanding of T-cell responses have helped shape our approach to the study of T cells in IBD. The notion put forward by Mosmann et al. that helper T cells can be distinguished based on cytokine profiles (ie, Th1 and Th2) [48,49] has led to the attempt to classify "immune" diseases (including CD and UC) into either Th1- or Th2-driven inflammatory processes. Indeed, CD – with its characteristic granulomas, the quintessential marker of a delayed-type hypersensitivity reaction, and the associated increases in interferon-γ and tumor necrosis factor (TNF)α – has been deemed a Th1 disease. UC, on the other hand, has been categorized on the Th2 side of the spectrum, although the evidence that UC patients have increased levels of IL-4 has not been well substantiated.

While it is clear that this basic dichotomy of T-cell function is an over-simplification, this model has provided a framework with which to explore the role of T cells in the immunopathogenesis of IBD. In one elegant study, both Th1 and Th2 T-cell clones were shown to individually drive intestinal inflammation in response to a bacterially derived antigen. The intestinal pathology initiated in this model showed that Th1 T cells led to a CD-like pathology, while Th2-driven colitis mimicked that seen in UC [50].

The study of different cytokine profiles in disease has led to the mapping of a complex network of cytokine pathways involved in IBD; some possibly involved in the initiation and/or perpetuation of the immune response, and others secondarily influenced by the inflammatory process. Dissecting this complex network may well require new informatic technologies based on artificial intelligence. Nonetheless, a select number of cytokines have led to potential new therapeutic targets. The success of the anti-TNFα monoclonal antibody, infliximab, and its successors are prime examples [51]. On the other hand, use of recombinant IL-10, a cytokine with potent immunoregulatory function, failed to provide clinical benefit in large randomized clinical trials [52,53]. This experience highlights the need to redefine our experimental findings based on clinical experience.

Regulatory T cells

An exciting development in the understanding of immune networks is a resurgence of interest in what used to be called "T suppressor" cells and are now more correctly referred to as "regulatory T cells" (Treg). Although it has always been assumed that the homeostasis of any biologic system, such as the immune response, requires checks and balances, the identification of T cells with the ability to regulate immune reactivity has only recently been well defined. Much of this work was developed in *in vivo* animal experiments, such as models of oral tolerance [54,55]. Work exploring the mouse model of CD45RBhi-induced colitis led to the observation that CD45RBlo T cells confer protection against CD45RBhi T-cell-induced colitis in recipient severe combined immunodeficiency (SCID) mice [56,57]. These findings led to the phenotypic identification of a subset of Treg-bearing CD45RBlo or CD25 markers. Subsequent studies identified IL-10 and transforming growth factor-β as mediators of Treg function. As might be expected, several phenotypically different Treg cells are now known, each identified in a different model system. Some of these do not depend on cytokine mediators, but instead work through cell–cell contact [58–61]. Some Treg cells are naturally occurring, while others are inducible or function to mediate oral tolerance [62]. The exact relationship between these different Treg cells continues to evolve [63]. More importantly, the human equivalent Treg cell and its potential role in IBD remain to be defined [64].

The presence of such Treg cells would suggest a potential therapeutic strategy directed at altering the underlying immune disease; however, while Treg cells or any immune manipulation work well in preventing inflammation in animal models of colitis, inflammation has been difficult to reverse once initiated. In one study, interfering with CD40/CD40-ligand interactions prevented

CD45RBhi colitis [65]. More recently, CD25 T cells administered to mice undergoing CD45RBhi-induced colitis reversed the intestinal inflammation [66]. These observations now suggest that a strategy targeted at manipulating the immune response in patients with established IBD can be developed.

Therefore, the Th1–Th2 paradigm does not completely explain the different animal models of colitis or the human disease accurately, but has provided a framework for understanding alterations in immune function. It appears that immune defects fall into either excessive effector T-cell function or defective regulatory T-cell function (see **Table 1**) [32]. How will this alter our understanding and possibly our treatment of patients with IBD? As mentioned, CD25 T cells can ameliorate colitis 4 weeks after onset. This allows for the possibility that appropriate use of regulatory T cells may offer a therapeutic option for patients with established IBD. We have recently shown that, by using an ovalbumin (OVA)-specific TCR transgenic mouse as the source of CD45RBhi T cells for transfer into SCID mice, we could induce Treg function by feeding the recipient mice OVA and prevent the development of colitis [67]. This observation suggests that the antigen specificity of the Treg cell does not restrict its function to T cells sharing antigen specificity, and opens up new strategies to activate Treg cells *in vivo*.

Lessons from studies of host–microbe interactions

Studies of the microbial interactions involved in IBD are well reviewed by Elson and Cong [68]. The hypothesis that gut bacterial flora contribute to IBD has been supported by observations both in animal models and in humans. CD patients with intestinal diversion undergo clinical and endoscopic remission. Once the gut is reanastomosed or the gut contents are reinstilled into the distal limb, inflammation resumes [69]. As mentioned, the presence of gut flora is required for the initiation of intestinal inflammation in most animal models. Whether this reactivity to bacteria represents a specific (ie, T-cell

Animal model	Epithelium	Innate immunity	T-cell activation	Regulatory T cells	B-cell activation
Dextran sulfate	+				
TNBS	+			+	
N-cadherin deficient	+				
Mdr-1 deficient	+				
Trefoil factor deficient	+				
Anti-CD3			+	?	
SEB			+		
TCRα deficient			?	+	+
C.rodentium			+		
Enterohepatic Helicobacter spp.		+	?		
C3H/HeJ-Bir			+		
CD45RBhi-SCID			+	+	
IL-10 deficient	+			+	
IL-2 deficient			+	+	

Table 1. Mechanistic defect or alteration associated with different animal models of intestinal inflammation. A cross (+) indicates where the defect/alteration acts on the model; a blank cell indicates a possible area of action; a question mark (?) indicates that no data are available. IL: interleukin; mdr: multidrug resistance gene; SCID: severe combined immunodeficiency; SEB: staphylococcal enterotoxin B; TCR: T-cell receptor; TNBS: trinitrobenzoic sulfate.

mediated), nonspecific, or innate immune response is the focus of intense investigation.

In a mouse model of *Citrobacter rodentium* infection, colitis was shown to be initiated by a bacteria-driven Th1 response that is not necessarily dependent on antigen-specific recognition [70]. In another model, bacteria-reactive T cells from colitic C3H/HEJ-Bir mice transferred colitis to recipient mice, and those T cells appeared to react specifically to cecal bacterial antigen components [71]. Thus, bacteria-reactive T cells can induce colitis. On the other hand, there appears to be a role for the innate immune system. Two recent studies have tried to tease apart the possibility that the innate immune response to enteric microbes can contribute to colitis. These have indicated that Treg cells may indeed alter the reactivity of the innate immune response against pathogenic and nonpathogenic microbes [72,73].

The search for an identifiable microbe that might account for either the initiation or perpetuation of disease has been unsuccessful. The examination of individual strains of enteric flora has identified a number of bacteria, many of which are constituents of the normal enteric flora, that may contribute to inflammation in an appropriate host [74,75]. Work using laser capture microscopy has demonstrated the intriguing finding of *Mycobacterium paratuberculosis* DNA, identified by polymerase chain reaction (PCR), on granulomas microscopically dissected out of CD tissue [76] – although the nonspecificity of this very sensitive technique may influence such results. Whether this means that *Mycobacterium* is the cause of CD or not, it certainly illustrates how difficult it is to be sure that we are using the correct technology when searching for a microbial etiology. We have recently examined colonoscopic biopsies from a cohort of IBD patients and controls for PCR-amplified *Helicobacter* ribosomal DNA sequences. The results of this study showed that *Helicobacter* DNA was identified in a significantly greater number of UC patients than either controls or CD patients. The sequencing of these PCR-amplified products suggests stronger homology with *H.pylori* than with either *H.bilis* or *H.hepaticus* [77].

Conclusion

The pathogenesis of CD and UC remains a mystery. Neither an etiologic microbe nor an immune defect that accounts for either CD or UC has been identified. A gene mutation has been identified that is associated with a very high risk of developing CD, but the explanation as to how this mutation leads to intestinal inflammation has remained elusive. Yet our understanding of the basic mechanisms of barrier function, immune regulation, and bacteria–host interactions has increased in leaps and bounds. We now understand that there is a need to improve the way in which studies of microbe–enteric flora interactions with the host are approached – taking advantage of advances in cellular and molecular tools to analyze immune function, using gnotobiotic facilities, and developing a greater understanding of the interactions between bacteria (eg, probiotics versus pathogenic bacteria).

The scientific community is poised to take advantage of a large number of advances in our understanding of numerous cellular processes (including cell activation, cell death and apoptosis, cell trafficking, cytokine networks, and mechanisms of tissue damage) to develop targets for new biologics. The real challenge for the next several years will be to understand how these elements can be manipulated to alter the natural history of CD and UC and develop therapeutic maneuvers that offer IBD patients the hope of a cure.

Acknowledgments

The author's research has been funded by the Crohn's and Colitis Foundation of Canada (CCFC), the Medical Research Council of Canada, Canadian Institutes of Health Research, and the Canadian Association of Gastroenterology, and the author has held an Ontario Ministry of Health Research Scientist Award. The author is currently the holder of a CCFC IBD Research Scientist Award.

References

1. Sutherland LR, Ramcharan S, Bryant H, et al. Effect of cigarette smoking on recurrence of Crohn's disease. *Gastroenterology* 1990;98:1123–8.
2. Levenstein S, Prantera C, Varvo V, et al. Stress and exacerbation in ulcerative colitis: a prospective study of patients enrolled in remission. *Am J Gastroenterol* 2000;95:1213–20.
3. Sandborn WJ, Tremaine WJ, Offord KP, et al. Transdermal nicotine for mildly to moderately active ulcerative colitis. A randomized, double-blind, placebo-controlled trial. *Ann Intern Med* 1997;126:364–71.
4. Jani N, Regueiro MD. Medical therapy for ulcerative colitis. *Gastroenterol Clin North Am* 2002;31:147–66.
5. Sonnenberg A, Cucino C, Bauerfeind P. Commentary: the unresolved mystery of birth-cohort phenomena in gastroenterology. *Int J Epidemiol* 2002;31:23–6.
6. Delco F, Sonnenberg A. Birth-cohort phenomenon in the time trends of mortality from ulcerative colitis. *Am J Epidemiol* 1999;150:359–66.
7. Delco F, Sonnenberg A. Commonalities in the time trends of Crohn's disease and ulcerative colitis. *Am J Gastroenterol* 1999;94:2171–6.
8. Radford-Smith GL, Edwards JE, Purdie DM, et al. Protective role of appendicectomy on onset and severity of ulcerative colitis and Crohn's disease. *Gut* 2002;51:808–13.
9. Sachar DB. Appendix redux. *Gut* 2002;51:764–5.
10. Mizoguchi A, Mizoguchi E, Chiba C, et al. Role of appendix in the development of inflammatory bowel disease in TCR-alpha mutant mice. *J Exp Med* 1996;184:707–15.
11. Hampe J, Cuthbert A, Croucher PJ, et al. Association between insertion mutation in NOD2 gene and Crohn's disease in German and British populations. *Lancet* 2001;357:1925–8.
12. Ogura Y, Bonen DK, Inohara N, et al. A frameshift mutation in NOD2 associated with susceptibility to Crohn's disease. *Nature* 2001;411:603–6.
13. Hugot JP, Chamaillard M, Zouali H, et al. Association of NOD2 leucine-rich repeat variants with susceptibility to Crohn's disease. *Nature* 2001;411:599–603.
14. Girardin SE, Hugot JP, Sansonetti PJ. Lessons from Nod2 studies: towards a link between Crohn's disease and bacterial sensing. *Trends Immunol* 2003;24:652–8.
15. Girardin SE, Travassos LH, Herve M, et al. Peptidoglycan molecular requirements allowing detection by Nod1 and Nod2. *J Biol Chem* 2003;278:41702–8.
16. Inohara N, Nunez G. NODs: intracellular proteins involved in inflammation and apoptosis. *Nat Rev Immunol* 2003;3:371–82.
17. Brant SR, Picco MF, Achkar JP, et al. Defining complex contributions of NOD2/CARD15 gene mutations, age at onset, and tobacco use on Crohn's disease phenotypes. *Inflamm Bowel Dis* 2003;9:281–9.
18. Helio T, Halme L, Lappalainen M, et al. CARD15/NOD2 gene variants are associated with familially occurring and complicated forms of Crohn's disease. *Gut* 2003;52:558–62.
19. Louis E, Michel V, Hugot JP, et al. Early development of stricturing or penetrating pattern in Crohn's disease is influenced by disease location, number of flares, and smoking but not by NOD2/CARD15 genotype. *Gut* 2003;52:552–7.
20. Cuthbert AP, Fisher SA, Mirza MM, et al. The contribution of NOD2 gene mutations to the risk and site of disease in inflammatory bowel disease. *Gastroenterology* 2002;122:867–74.

21. Abreu MT, Taylor KD, Lin YC, et al. Mutations in NOD2 are associated with fibrostenosing disease in patients with Crohn's disease. *Gastroenterology* 2002;123:679–88.

22. Aldhous MC, Nimmo ER, Satsangi J. NOD2/CARD15 and the Paneth cell: another piece in the genetic jigsaw of inflammatory bowel disease. *Gut* 2003;52:1533–5.

23. Ogura Y, Lala S, Xin W, et al. Expression of NOD2 in Paneth cells: a possible link to Crohn's ileitis. *Gut* 2003;52:1591–7.

24. Lala S, Ogura Y, Osborne C, et al. Crohn's disease and the NOD2 gene: a role for paneth cells. *Gastroenterology* 2003;125:47–57.

25. Erdman S, Fox JG, Dangler CA, et al. Typhlocolitis in NF-kappa B-deficient mice. *J Immunol* 2001;166:1443–7.

26. Negoro K, McGovern DP, Kinouchi Y, et al. Analysis of the IBD5 locus and potential gene–gene interactions in Crohn's disease. *Gut* 2003;52:541–6.

27. Mombaerts P, Mizoguchi E, Grusby MJ, et al. Spontaneous development of inflammatory bowel disease in T cell receptor mutant mice. *Cell* 1993;75:275–82.

28. Kuhn R, Lohler J, Rennick D, et al. Interleukin-10-deficient mice develop chronic enterocolitis. *Cell* 1993;75:263–74.

29. Sadlack B, Merz H, Schorle H, et al. Ulcerative colitis-like disease in mice with a disrupted interleukin-2 gene. *Cell* 1993;75:253–61.

30. Bouma G, Strober W. The immunological and genetic basis of inflammatory bowel disease. *Nat Rev Immunol* 2003;3:521–33.

31. Pizarro TT, Arseneau KO, Bamias G, et al. Mouse models for the study of Crohn's disease. *Trends Mol Med* 2003;9:218–22.

32. Strober W, Fuss IJ, Blumberg RS. The immunology of mucosal models of inflammation. *Annu Rev Immunol* 2002;20:495–549.

33. Irvine EJ, Marshall JK. Increased intestinal permeability precedes the onset of Crohn's disease in a subject with familial risk. *Gastroenterology* 2000;119:1740–4.

34. Meddings J. Barrier dysfunction and Crohn's disease. *Ann NY Acad Sci* 2000;915:333–8.

35. Hermiston ML, Gordon JI. Inflammatory bowel disease and adenomas in mice expressing a dominant negative N-cadherin. *Science* 1995;270:1203–7.

36. Podolsky DK. Mechanisms of regulatory peptide action in the gastrointestinal tract: trefoil peptides. *J Gastroenterol* 2000;35(Suppl. 12):69–74.

37. L'Heureux MC, Brubaker PL. Therapeutic potential of the intestinotropic hormone, glucagon-like peptide-2. *Ann Med* 2001;33:229–35.

38. Tsai CH, Hill M, Asa SL, et al. Intestinal growth-promoting properties of glucagon-like peptide-2 in mice. *Am J Physiol* 1997;273:E77–84.

39. Panwala CM, Jones JC, Viney JL. A novel model of inflammatory bowel disease: mice deficient for the multiple drug resistance gene, *mdr1a*, spontaneously develop colitis. *J Immunol* 1998;161:5733–44.

40. Maggio-Price L, Shows D, Waggie K, et al. *Helicobacter bilis* infection accelerates and *H. hepaticus* infection delays the development of colitis in multiple drug resistance-deficient (mdr1a–/–) mice. *Am J Pathol* 2002;160:739–51.

41. Sandborn WJ, Loftus EV Jr, Colombel JF, et al. Evaluation of serologic disease markers in a population-based cohort of patients with ulcerative colitis and Crohn's disease. *Inflamm Bowel Dis* 2001;7:192–201.

42. Bernstein CN, Orr K, Blanchard JF, et al. Development of an assay for antibodies to *Saccharomyces cerevisiae*: Easy, cheap and specific for Crohn's disease. *Can J Gastroenterol* 2001;15:499–504.

43. Dubinsky MC, Ofman JJ, Urman M, et al. Clinical utility of serodiagnostic testing in suspected pediatric inflammatory bowel disease. *Am J Gastroenterol* 2001;96:758–65.

44. Wei B, Huang T, Dalwadi H, et al. *Pseudomonas fluorescens* encodes the Crohn's disease-associated I2 sequence and T-cell superantigen. *Infect Immun* 2002;70:6567–75.

45. Dalwadi H, Wei B, Kronenberg M, et al. The Crohn's disease-associated bacterial protein I2 is a novel enteric T cell superantigen. *Immunity* 2001;15:149–58.

46. Landers CJ, Cohavy O, Misra R, et al. Selected loss of tolerance evidenced by Crohn's disease-associated immune responses to auto- and microbial antigens. *Gastroenterology* 2002;123:689–99.

47. Mizoguchi E, Mizoguchi A, Preffer FI, et al. Regulatory role of mature B cells in a murine model of inflammatory bowel disease. *Int Immunol* 2000;12:597–605.

48. Mosmann TR, Cherwinski H, Bond MW, et al. Two types of murine helper T cell clone. I. Definition according to profiles of lymphokine activities and secreted proteins. *J Immunol* 1986;136:2348–57.

49. Schaible UE, Kramer MD, Museteanu C, et al. The severe combined immunodeficiency (*scid*) mouse. A laboratory model for the analysis of Lyme arthritis and carditis. *J Exp Med* 1989;170:1427–32.

50. Iqbal N, Oliver JR, Wagner FH, et al. T helper 1 and T helper 2 cells are pathogenic in an antigen-specific model of colitis. *J Exp Med* 2002;195:71–84.

51. Targan SR, Hanauer SB, Van Deventer SJ, et al. A short-term study of chimeric monoclonal antibody cA2 to tumor necrosis factor alpha for Crohn's disease. Crohn's Disease cA2 Study Group. *N Engl J Med* 1997;337:1029–35.

52. Fedorak RN, Gangl A, Elson CO, et al. Recombinant human interleukin 10 in the treatment of patients with mild to moderately active Crohn's disease. The Interleukin 10 Inflammatory Bowel Disease Cooperative Study Group. *Gastroenterology* 2000;119:1473–82.

53. Schreiber S, Fedorak RN, Nielsen OH, et al. Safety and efficacy of recombinant human interleukin 10 in chronic active Crohn's disease. Crohn's Disease IL-10 Cooperative Study Group. *Gastroenterology* 2000;119:1461–72.

54. Khoury SJ, Hancock WW, Weiner HL. Oral tolerance to myelin basic protein and natural recovery from experimental autoimmune encephalomyelitis are associated with downregulation of inflammatory cytokines and differential upregulation of transforming growth factor beta, interleukin 4, and prostaglandin E expression in the brain. *J Exp Med* 1992;176:1355–64.

55. Miller A, Lider O, Weiner HL. Antigen-driven bystander suppression after oral administration of antigens. *J Exp Med* 1991;174:791–8.

56. Powrie F, Leach MW, Mauze S, et al. Phenotypically distinct subsets of CD4+ T cells induce or protect from chronic intestinal inflammation in C. B-17 scid mice. *Int Immunol* 1993;5:1461–71.

57. Morrissey PJ, Charrier K, Braddy S, et al. CD4+ T cells that express high levels of CD45RB induce wasting disease when transferred into congenic severe combined immunodeficient mice. Disease development is prevented by cotransfer of purified CD4+ T cells. *J Exp Med* 1993;178:237–44.

58. Thornton AM, Shevach EM. CD4+CD25+ immunoregulatory T cells suppress polyclonal T cell activation *in vitro* by inhibiting interleukin 2 production. *J Exp Med* 1998;188:287–96.

59. Fuss IJ, Boirivant M, Lacy B, et al. The interrelated roles of TGF-beta and IL-10 in the regulation of experimental colitis. *J Immunol* 2002;168:900–8.

60. Nakamura K, Kitani A, Strober W. Cell contact-dependent immunosuppression by CD4(+)CD25(+) regulatory T cells is mediated by cell surface-bound transforming growth factor beta. *J Exp Med* 2001;194:629–44.

61. Strober W, Kelsall B, Fuss I, et al. Reciprocal IFN-gamma and TGF-beta responses regulate the occurrence of mucosal inflammation. *Immunol Today* 1997;18:61–4.

15

62. Weiner HL. Oral tolerance, an active immunologic process mediated by multiple mechanisms. *J Clin Invest* 2000;106:935–7.

63. Toms C, Powrie F. Control of intestinal inflammation by regulatory T cells. *Microbes Infect* 2001;3:929–35.

64. Azuma T, Takahashi T, Kunisato A, et al. Human CD4+ CD25+ regulatory T cells suppress NKT cell functions. *Cancer Res* 2003;63:4516–20.

65. Liu Z, Geboes K, Colpaert S, et al. Prevention of experimental colitis in SCID mice reconstituted with CD45RBhigh CD4+ T cells by blocking the CD40–CD154 interactions. *J Immunol* 2000;164:6005–14.

66. Mottet C, Uhlig HH, Powrie F. Cutting edge: cure of colitis by CD4(+)CD25(+) regulatory T cells. *J Immunol* 2003;170:3939–43.

67. Zhou P, Borojevic R, Streutker C, et al. Expression of dual T cell receptor on DO11.10 T cells allows for OVA-induced oral tolerance to prevent T cell mediated colitis directed against unrelated enteric bacterial antigens. *J Immunol* 2004;172:1515–23.

68. Elson CO, Cong Y. Understanding immune-microbial homeostasis in intestine. *Immunol Res* 2002;26:87–94.

69. D'Haens GR, Geboes K, Peeters M, et al. Early lesions of recurrent Crohn's disease caused by infusion of intestinal contents in excluded ileum. *Gastroenterology* 1998;114:262–7.

70. Higgins LM, Frankel G, Douce G, et al. *Citrobacter rodentium* infection in mice elicits a mucosal Th1 cytokine response and lesions similar to those in murine inflammatory bowel disease. *Infect Immun* 1999;67:3031–9.

71. Cong Y, Brandwein SL, McCabe RP, et al. CD4+ T cells reactive to enteric bacterial antigens in spontaneously colitic C3H/HeJBir mice: Increased T helper cell type 1 response and ability to transfer disease. *J Exp Med* 1998;187:855–64.

72. Maloy KJ, Salaun L, Cahill R, et al. CD4+CD25+ T(R) cells suppress innate immune pathology through cytokine-dependent mechanisms. *J Exp Med* 2003;197:111–19.

73. Kullberg MC, Jankovic D, Gorelick PL, et al. Bacteria-triggered CD4(+) T regulatory cells suppress *Helicobacter hepaticus*-induced colitis. *J Exp Med* 2002;196:505–15.

74. Jiang HQ, Kushnir N, Thurnheer MC, et al. Monoassociation of SCID mice with *Helicobacter muridarum*, but not four other enterics, provokes IBD upon receipt of T cells. *Gastroenterology* 2002;122:1346–54.

75. Rath HC, Schultz M, Freitag R, et al. Different subsets of enteric bacteria induce and perpetuate experimental colitis in rats and mice. *Infect Immun* 2001;69:2277–85.

76. Ryan P, Bennett MW, Aarons S, et al. PCR detection of *Mycobacterium paratuberculosis* in Crohn's disease granulomas isolated by laser capture microdissection. *Gut* 2002;51:665–70.

77. Streutker CJ, Bernstein CN, Chan VL, et al. Detection of species-specific helicobacter ribosomal DNA in intestinal biopsies from a population-based cohort of patients with ulcerative colitis. *J Clin Microbiol* 2004;42:660–4.

2

Clinical, molecular, and serological subtyping of the manifestations of Crohn's disease

Ian DR Arnott and Jack Satsangi

Introduction

Since Crohn and Ginzberg's description of an inflammatory and stricturing disease of the terminal ileum in 1932 [1], phenotypic, serologic, and molecular heterogeneity have been increasingly recognized within the diagnosis of Crohn's disease (CD). There has been an effort to categorize the observed variability; this was initially driven by a wish to individualize treatment and to understand the role of serological markers in inflammatory bowel disease (IBD), but also more recently by progress in understanding the molecular genetics of CD. Animal models of colitis have demonstrated that a number of different genetic and environmental influences can result in gastrointestinal inflammation, signifying a final common pathway [2]. The identification of phenotypic subcategories may lead to the detection of a related group of gastrointestinal illnesses, rather than a single condition called CD.

In this chapter, we document recent advances in the clinical and molecular methods that are available to classify CD, and discuss the implications for stratification of treatment and elucidation of the pathogenesis of this disease.

Classification of the clinical manifestations of CD

Initial classifications of the clinical manifestations of CD focused on establishing robust criteria for the diagnosis of IBD. Lennard-

Jones divided inflammation within the bowel into that with a known cause, most commonly an infectious etiology, and that without a known cause. These criteria, which were established for the diagnosis of CD and ulcerative colitis (UC), remain highly relevant to IBD research today [3].

Anatomical location

The first attempts to classify the manifestations of CD were based on anatomical location of disease. Farmer et al. subdivided anatomical involvement into ileal alone, ileocolonic, colonic alone, and anal/perianal [4]. Of 615 patients assessed, ileocolonic disease was present in 252 (41%) patients, the small intestine (ileal alone) was involved in 176 (29%), colonic disease in 166 (27%), and anorectal disease in 21 (3%). Long-term follow-up of these patients found the location of disease to be relatively stable after 10 years [5]. The investigators found that both the symptoms and the complications of the disease varied between subdivisions. These subdivisions have subsequently been found to be of relevance in terms of medical therapy [6], indications for surgery [5], and risk of postoperative recurrence in childhood [7].

Disease behavior

Further attempts at subdivision focused on disease behavior, an area where disease heterogeneity is most manifest. CD disease behavior was initially described as either perforating or nonperforating as an indication for surgery. Greenstein et al. found that reoperation was required twice as quickly when there was a perforating indication for the initial operation [8]. This was seen across all anatomical distributions and for second to third operations, as well as for first to second. Disease behavior was then extrapolated to define three subtypes – inflammatory, stricturing, and penetrating disease – which were encompassed in the Rome classification [9]. These features were not mutually exclusive and subdivision proved difficult; the classification could potentially result in 756 individual phenotypes and yielded only moderate interobserver correlation [10]. This classification was therefore not widely adopted.

The clinical relevance of the division of disease behavior has also been the subject of some debate. Analyzing 101 CD patients, Aeberhard et al. found that the only clinical feature that related to the speed of operation was whether the disease was perforating or nonperforating. The median time to a second operation was 1.7 years for perforating disease versus 13 years for nonperforating disease [11]. Analysis of our own cohort of Vienna-classified patients (see below) found similar results, with highest operation rates in penetrating disease. We also found significantly higher rates of surgery in stricturing disease than in inflammatory disease [12]. This has not, however, been confirmed by other groups, who did not identify differences between operation rates in those with perforating and nonperforating disease [13,14].

The Vienna classification
In 1996, an international working party was established to develop a simple, objective, and reproducible classification of CD. Following five meetings over the next 2 years, the Vienna classification was developed and finally published in 2000 [15]. This classification divides CD according to three overriding clinical variables:

- patient age at diagnosis

- location of disease

- disease behavior

Age at diagnosis is divided into <40 years (A1) and >40 years (A2). Location of disease is defined as the maximal extent of disease prior to the first surgery, and is subdivided into terminal ileum (L1), colon (L2), ileocolon (L3), and upper gastrointestinal tract (L4). Disease behavior is divided by a hierarchical system into mutually exclusive groups comprising inflammatory (B1), stricturing (B2), and penetrating (B3) disease. The Vienna classification is outlined in **Table 1**. This

Age at diagnosis	A1	<40 years
	A2	>40 years
Disease location	L1	Terminal ileum
	L2	Colon
	L3	Ileocolon
	L4	Upper gastrointestinal tract
Disease behavior	B1	Inflammatory (nonstricturing, nonpenetrating)
	B2	Stricturing
	B3	Penetrating

Table 1. The Vienna classification of Crohn's disease.

classification has been shown to give good interobserver correlation [16] and has now been adopted more widely [17,18].

It is the subgroup of disease behavior that has attracted much recent interest. Three studies have examined the stability of disease phenotype over time and the factors that influence progression from one phenotype to another. It is now clear that although disease location is relatively stable over time (differing significantly 10 years following diagnosis [18]), disease behavior is not. Louis et al. examined the stability of phenotype in a Belgian population of CD patients who were followed for up to 25 years [18]. Striking changes in disease behavior were noted over time: within 10 years, the disease behavior of 46% of patients had changed from purely inflammatory disease to either stricturing or penetrating disease. Relative to this finding, disease location was stable, although this had also changed in approximately 15% of patients by 10 years. It was thought that disease behavior assessed at a single time point was likely to be a poor phenotypic marker in genotype/phenotype analyses.

In the largest study to date, Cosnes et al. retrospectively analyzed data concerning the long-term evolution of disease behavior in 2,002 CD patients, and performed a 5-year prospective analysis on a subgroup of 646 patients [14]. After 20 years, 88% of the initial inflammatory disease cohort had developed either stricturing (18%) or penetrating (70%) disease behavior. In this study, disease location was identified as the most important factor in determining an alteration in disease behavior, with small bowel and anoperineal involvement predicting early stricturing and/or penetrating complications. More recently, Louis et al. examined in detail the factors that may influence disease progression in a cohort of 163 patients followed for 5 years from diagnosis [19]. A total of 32.5% of patients with inflammatory disease at diagnosis progressed to a more severe phenotype over 5 years. The major determinants of progression were disease location and the number of flares per year: ileal location of the disease was associated with a stricturing pattern, while a high number of flares was associated with a penetrating pattern.

The above studies have demonstrated that the natural history of CD involves progression to a more complicated disease type. Although analysis has demonstrated that this progression is related to anatomical location of disease, the factors governing the speed of progression are poorly characterized. We have subsequently analyzed a cohort of 142 CD patients with regard to disease progression [12]. As in the above studies, we found disease location to be a major determinant of disease behavior, with 35% of patients with ileal disease having stricturing or penetrating disease at diagnosis compared with only 17% of patients with isolated colonic disease. In addition, we found a strong relationship between progression and the presence of anti-*Saccharomyces cerevisiae* antibody (ASCA) (at 5 years, disease progressed in 54% of ASCA-positive patients versus 21% of ASCA-negative patients) and a relatively protective effect of variant *NOD2/CARD15* alleles.

There remain a number of difficulties with the Vienna classification, notably the uncertain stability over time of disease behavior and, to a lesser extent, location. Some also feel that the inclusion of perianal disease as penetrating disease may not be appropriate. The presence of perianal disease is independent of the behavior of intestinal disease [20], and the classification of disease behavior as penetrating disease may deflect attention away from the individual's predominant problem. For example, a patient may have relatively mild perianal disease but a tight and troublesome ileal stricture – under the Vienna classification, they would be classified as having penetrating disease. Nevertheless, the Vienna classification remains the most reproducible classification of CD available at present, and its use will help to strengthen both clinical studies and those relating to pathogenesis. It is, however, the limitations of the clinical classifications together with the inherent heterogeneity of CD that have stimulated a further search for and analysis of subclinical markers of CD.

Subclinical divisions of CD

Genetic markers

While the etiology of CD remains unknown, it is now clear that gene–environment interactions are central to understanding the disease pathogenesis. Clear evidence for a strong genetic component to CD is available, most notably through concordance rates in twins and other first- and second-degree relatives. Moreover, clinical data suggest that not only disease susceptibility, but also phenotypic characteristics, have a genetic basis.

The presence of a genetic component of disease raises the question as to whether the phenotype of familial disease differs from that of sporadic CD. Some studies, but not others, have found the age at onset and age at diagnosis to be younger in those with familial disease [21]. Younger age at diagnosis has also been associated with more ileal disease, more stricturing disease, and surgery for intractable disease. Older age has been associated with more colonic disease and inflammatory disease behavior [22]. There is no consistent difference in disease location and disease behavior between familial and sporadic CD [21].

A series of genetic markers that may determine susceptibility/ phenotype have been proposed, of which the most promising are those within regions of linkage (susceptibility loci). These putative candidate genes have been identified by the parallel techniques of genome-wide scanning and positional candidate gene analysis [23].

NOD2/CARD15

Detailed evaluation of the susceptibility locus on chromosome 16 has led to the identification of the *IBD1* gene as *NOD2/CARD15* [24,25]. *NOD2/CARD15* contains a highly conserved caspase recruitment domain (CARD) linked to a nucleotide-binding oligomerization domain (NOD), which are thought to regulate apoptosis and nuclear factor-κB activation. The C-terminal domain of *NOD2/CARD15* comprises a leucine-rich repeat region, which has sequence homology with a number of plant disease resistance genes, and the toll and toll-like receptor gene superfamilies.

The contribution of *NOD2/CARD15* has been studied in many diverse populations [25–29], with positive associations in up to 50% of CD patients [30]. However, data from Japanese, Korean, and African-American individuals have not shown an association [2,31–33], and there are clear differences between Ashkenazi Jewish and non-Jewish populations [34,35]. Most recent data from Ireland and northern Europe report relatively low allelic frequencies in healthy controls and CD patients, and raise the possibility of heterogeneity within European populations of distinct ancestry [36–39].

Attempts to relate the *NOD2/CARD15* genotype to a phenotype have been confounded by the validity of subclassifications used [40], but it is apparent from a number of articles that genotype–phenotype relationships do exist. The phenotypic associations observed in individual studies are displayed in **Table 2**. The most consistently reported relationship of variant *NOD2/CARD15* alleles is with ileal disease [26–30,36–38,41],

Study	Phenotype				
	Early onset	Ileal disease	Disease type	Surgery	EIM
Abreu et al., 2002 [26]	No	Yes	Stricturing	ND	ND
Ahmad et al., 2002 [29]	Yes	Yes	Protective of penetrating	No	No
Bairead et al., 2003 [36]	Yes	Yes	ND	ND	ND
Cuthbert et al., 2002 [28]	ND	Yes	ND	ND	ND
Hampe et al., 2002 [37]	No	Yes	Stricturing	No	No
Helio et al., 2003 [38]	No	Yes	Stricturing and penetrating	Yes	ND
Lesage et al., 2002 [30]	Yes	Yes	Stricturing	No	No
Tomer et al., 2003 [41]	No	Yes	ND	No	No
Vermeire et al., 2002 [27]	No	Yes	No	No	No

Table 2. Phenotypic associations of variant *NOD2/CARD15* alleles. EIM: extraintestinal manifestations; ND: no data (analysis was not done or not reported on); No: no association was detected; Yes: a positive association was detected.

and the single-nucleotide polymorphism most commonly associated with this distribution is the frame-shift mutation [29,36]. There is now emerging evidence that this pattern of disease may be related to the distribution of Paneth cells within the gastrointestinal tract. These cells express NOD2/CARD15, are concentrated in the terminal ileum, and have a role in innate immunity via the secretion of defensins [43,44]. Smaller studies have not been able to confirm the association with ileal disease, presumably a type I error. There is also a gene-dosage effect; Lesage et al. suggested that patients carrying two variant copies of the *NOD2/CARD15* gene are at increased risk of ileal involvement [30]. This effect has also been identified by others [29,42] – indeed, in the study of Ahmad et al., 100% of homozygotes or compound heterozygotes had evidence of ileal involvement (not Vienna classified) [29].

Conversely, an inverse association of colonic disease with *NOD2/CARD15* has been identified [26–29,42]. This is consistent with recent data demonstrating the absense of NOD2/CARD15 protein [25,45] and Paneth cells from the colon (except in areas of metaplasia) [43].

Variant *NOD2/CARD15* alleles have also been associated with a fibrostenosing or stricturing disease type [26,29,30,42,46]. However, it is clear that ileal disease is strongly associated with stricturing disease type, regardless of *NOD2/CARD15* status [46]. In the analysis by Abreu et al., fibrostenosing behavior was seen as an independent variable in multivariate analysis [26], and this was confirmed in a subset analysis that stratified patients by the presence of small bowel disease. The study by Brant et al. identified both ileal disease and stricturing disease behavior as independent associations of *NOD2/CARD15* in a multivariate analysis [42]. This group used a modified Vienna classification scheme for the categorization of disease behavior. It is of interest that, under this system, which does not categorize perianal disease as penetrating disease, there was an association of penetrating disease and variant *NOD2/CARD15* alleles. One further study has identified this association, but classifications were not given [46]. Ahmad et al. also found an association between variant *NOD2/CARD15* alleles and fibrostenosing disease, but this was not independent of the association with ileal disease on multivariate analysis [29]. Others have been unable to confirm the association with stricturing disease, despite an association with ileal disease [27,28,36–38]. However, there does appear to be evidence that variant *NOD2/CARD15* alleles may be protective against the development of penetrating disease. Louis et al. did not observe any association between progression of disease type and *NOD2/CARD15* variants [19]. A re-examination of their data [47], together with data from our own unit [12] and from US and UK populations [26,29], would suggest that disease progression or the presence of penetrating disease is significantly lower in individuals carrying variant *NOD2/CARD15* alleles.

Variant *NOD2/CARD15* alleles have also been associated with early-onset disease [29,30,36] and, again, there may be a younger age of onset in patients carrying two variant alleles. This association has been more variably reported than the above, with many groups not observing the association [26–30,37,38], and recruitment bias of the studied populations should not be underestimated as a confounding factor. In a pediatric population, *NOD2/CARD15* has been associated with low birth weight of the patients [41].

The need for more frequent surgery has also been variably reported to be associated with variant *NOD2/CARD15* alleles [38,46], but again there is an association of frequent surgery with ileal disease and the primary association with genotype may be difficult to establish.

IBD3: HLA region
Despite strong evidence implicating immune dysfunction and genetic predisposition in the pathogenesis of CD, the overall importance of the genes of the major histocompatibility complex in susceptibility to CD remains uncertain, with conflicting evidence available. Population-based association studies of the human leukocyte antigen (HLA) region have had variable and inconclusive results for a number of reasons. Initial studies were carried out using serological typing, which is less reliable than the molecular typing that is currently available, and this has been compounded by difficulties with considerable ethnic and disease heterogeneity, together with problems of study power. A detailed early analysis

from Oxford of HLA-DRB1 and -DQB genes (class II determinants) revealed no association with CD susceptibility or disease behavior [48], although more recent data from the same center, and elsewhere in Europe, continue to implicate the class III region [49,50]. Association studies in homogeneous populations, such as the Japanese, have shown association [51], but analyses of more heterogeneous white populations have failed to demonstrate the link [48]. A meta-analysis of all available studies in 1999 demonstrated a positive association of CD and HLA-DR7 and -DRB*010, and a negative association of CD with HLA-DR2 and -DR3 [52]. These associations retained statistical significance, even when the homogeneous Japanese populations were removed from the analysis.

Studies assessing the phenotypic associations of *IBD3* in CD have shown positive but conflicting results. A study of HLA class I, HLA class II, and transporter associated with antigen processing (TAP) gene polymorphisms identified an association of HLA-DRB1*04 with glucocorticoid nonresponse, HLA-DQB1*0501 or -DQ5*0503 with the presence of extraintestinal manifestations, and HLA-DRB1*07 with small bowel disease [53]. There was no overall association of *TAP* genes with Crohn's disease, but variant *TAP2-A* alleles were more frequently found in patients who responded to corticosteroids. In a further study of Japanese patients, no overall association was observed between CD and HLA-B alleles, but there was an association of HLA-B alleles with isolated colonic disease in a subgroup genotype–phenotype analysis [54].

In the study by Ahmad et al., stronger evidence emerged for the association between HLA variants and CD phenotype [29]. HLA-DRB1*701 was associated with ileal disease, whereas the classic autoimmune haplotype HLA A1-B8-DR3 was associated with colonic disease. Some of the strongest links appeared to be with perianal disease, which was associated with the MICA*010 haplotype and DRB*0103. The latter was also associated with a penetrating disease type (which is closely linked to perianal disease).

Despite the variable associations documented above, firmer evidence exists for an association with the extraintestinal manifestations of CD. Orchard et al. found specific associations between type I arthropathy and HLA-DRB1*0103, -B*35, and -B*27, and type II arthropathy and HLA-B*44 [55]. The study group comprised a large cohort of IBD patients (483 CD, 976 UC) and there were no observable differences in the associations between CD and UC patients. This may illustrate the ability of individual genes to modify disease phenotype without conferring overall susceptibility. A subsequent analysis of this population found an association between ocular inflammation and HLA-B*27, -B*58, and -DRB1*0103. There was also a weak association between erythema nodosum and HLA-B*15. In addition, there was a strong association between the variant −1031 TNFα allele and erythema nodosum.

It is noteworthy that the association of *IBD3* and disease susceptibility is much stronger for UC, where it is estimated that the contribution of *IBD3* to overall genetic risk is 64%–100% (compared with a figure of 10%–33% for CD) [56]. Replicated phenotypic correlations have also been documented in UC, with DRB1*0103 being associated with extensive and severe colitis in white Europeans with CD [57], and DRB1*1502 being associated with extensive UC in Jewish [58] and Japanese populations [59].

IBD5

IBD5, located at chromosome 5q, was initially identified in a genome-wide scan of 158 Canadian families with IBD [60]. The association between the susceptibility locus 5q and CD has subsequently been replicated in other populations [61]. In the initial description, the association was of genome-wide significance only in families with early-onset disease (with at least one individual being diagnosed at age ≤16 years), suggesting a phenotypic association. However, subsequent studies of the index population and of other CD populations did not find any correlation between *IBD5* status and clinical manifestations of CD [27,62]. Further analysis of this locus by the

Oxford group has identified a phenotypic association: haplotype H2 was associated with perianal disease and ileal involvement [63]. The association between ileal disease and H2 was not seen in the absence of perianal disease, and a haplotype-dosage effect was observed.

Serological markers

The clarification of the pathogenic mechanisms of CD has highlighted the pivotal role that luminal bacteria play in perpetuating the inflammatory process. Animal model data have provided strong evidence for the role of enteric bacteria in intestinal inflammation: animal models of IBD develop colitis only in the presence of luminal bacteria [2,64]. In humans, diversion of the fecal stream has been shown to ameliorate colitis [65], and antibiotics and probiotics have had some success in IBD treatment [66–68].

As yet, there is no evidence of a specific pathogenic organism – indeed, most resident bacteria do not participate in the disease process [2] – but the recognition of muramyl dipeptide (MDP), a bacterial peptidoglycan motif [69], by NOD2 further implicates a role for bacteria in intestinal inflammation. It is clear, however, that the host's genetic background determines susceptibility to gut inflammation in individual mouse models [70].

Serological responses are well described in CD [71,72], although the diagnostic value and pathogenic importance of these serological markers are still under evaluation. Antibodies directed against the oligomannan component of *Saccharomyces cerevisiae* (ASCA) and the perinuclear component of neutrophils (pANCA) have been the most widely studied, and have been suggested to be of diagnostic importance in North American populations [73]. Antibodies against the outer-membrane porin protein C of *Escherichia coli* (anti-OmpC) and *Pseudomonas fluorescens* (anti-I2) have also been described in CD [71]. Many other antibody reactivities have been described in IBD, with over

	ASCA	pANCA	Anti-OmpC	Anti-I2
CD [73,76,78]	39–61	4–24	55	50
UC [73–77]	5–15	50–73	2	10
Healthy control	5	2.5	1.3	10

Table 3. Prevalence of antibodies against the oligomannan component of *Saccharomyces cerevisiae* (ASCA), the perinuclear component of neutrophils (pANCA), and the outer-membrane porin protein C of *Escherichia coli* (anti-OmpC) and *Pseudomonas fluorescens* (anti-I2) in Crohn's disease (CD), ulcerative colitis (UC), and controls. The figures presented are percentages. Comparative data for healthy controls come from our own unit.

22 main antibodies described [73]. Few, however, are assayed widely, even in the research environment.

ASCA has been observed in 39%–61% of CD patients [74,75] and 5%–15% of UC patients, whereas pANCA is present in 4%–24% of CD patients [76,77] and 50%–73% of UC patients [76,78]. In CD, reported seroprevalence is 55% for anti-OmpC and 50% for anti-I2 [71]. These antibodies are present in a small proportion of healthy control subjects and other forms of colonic disease [79,80]. Prevalence figures for these antibodies in CD, with comparative data from UC and healthy controls, are shown in **Table 3**.

ASCA has not realized its potential as a diagnostic marker as it lacks sufficient sensitivity and specificity. However, ASCA does have a role in differentiating CD from UC and accelerating diagnosis in patients with indeterminate colitis. There are also a number of phenotypic associations of ASCA, some of which may have implications for the pathogenesis of these antibodies. Phenotypic associations of ASCA are shown in **Table 4**.

The strongest phenotypic associations of ASCA in CD are with small bowel disease and a low incidence of colonic disease [81,82]. In one study, the prevalence of ASCA was 70% in

Clinical feature	Reference
Young age at diagnosis	75, 95, 96
Small bowel disease	81, 82, 96
Fibrostenosing disease	81, 95
No relationship to disease activity	71, 75, 82

Table 4. The phenotypic associations of ASCA.

patients with small bowel involvement compared with 46% in those with purely colonic disease [75]. ASCA has also been associated with early-onset CD [75], together with fibrostenosing and penetrating disease types [81,83] and multiple bowel surgery. We have also recently described a strong association between ASCA and progression of disease type from purely inflammatory disease to stricturing or penetrating disease [12].

pANCA in CD has been associated with a UC-like phenotype [81,84]. Vasiliauskas et al. examined 69 patients with CD and found 55% to be pANCA positive [81]. These patients were more likely to have left-sided colonic disease that was clinically reflected by rectal bleeding, mucus discharge, and the use of enemas as treatment. This was confirmed in a subsequent study [84], but others have been unable to confirm this finding [85]. A recent analysis of pANCA and ASCA according to the Vienna classification found late-onset disease (A2) to be associated with pANCA (19% vs 5% in A1 patients) [86]. pANCA was also associated with inflammatory disease type and ASCA was associated with upper gastrointestinal disease (L4) (positive in 66.7%). There are also provocative data to suggest that ASCA may be a subclinical marker of individuals at high risk for developing CD [87,88].

Recent evidence examining the antibodies anti-OmpC and anti-I2 in CD has identified novel associations. Data from a US population have demonstrated that the loss of tolerance to these antigens is not global, but rather is specific to individual microbial antigens, and stratification of patients based on the number and level of these antibody responses has now been demonstrated [71]. Multivariate analysis of a US population has found anti-OmpC to be associated with perforating disease type and anti-I2 to be associated with fibrostenosing disease and the need for small bowel surgery [89]. Complementary data from a European population, using the Vienna classification, found independent associations of anti-OmpC with progression of disease type and long disease duration and of anti-I2 with long disease duration and the need for surgery (IDR Arnott, manuscript submitted). Data from both populations have confirmed that the presence and magnitude of response to all studied microbial antigens is critical in determining disease phenotype. In both studies, patients with a higher cumulative number of responses and a greater total response to microbial antigens had a severe form of CD that was characterized by small bowel involvement and the need for intestinal surgery. This is illustrated by the data on disease progression and need for surgery. Disease progressed in 12.5% of patients who had total antibody responses in the lowest third of the cohort compared with 80% of patients with responses in the highest third. Similarly, 23% of patients with responses in the lowest third required surgery compared with 80% with responses in the highest third.

A number of findings differed between the two studies, possibly due to the different disease classifications used. The US cohort found the presence and magnitude of response to microbial antigens to be associated with fibrostenosing disease and intestinal perforation, while the European cohort identified associations with frequent disease progression and long disease duration. These findings have been reinforced in both cohorts by the use of cluster analysis, a technique that identifies groups of individuals with responses at the high end of the spectrum. A graphical representation of the clusters identified in the study by Landers et al. is displayed in **Figure 1** [71]. It is of great interest that despite demonstrable differences in the clinical

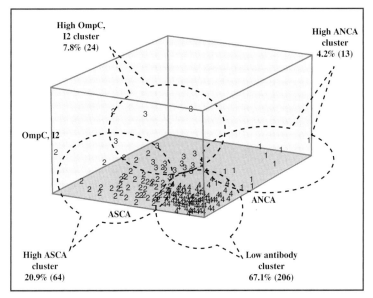

Figure 1. Three-dimensional scatterplot of the four clusters represented by high anti-neutrophil cytoplasmic antibody (ANCA), high anti-*Saccharomyces cerevisiae* antibody (ASCA) immunoglobulin (Ig)A and IgG, high anti-OmpC and anti-I2, and low values of all five antibodies. To represent the five antibodies in this figure, the average of ASCA IgA and ASCA IgG is plotted on the *x*-axis, the average of anti-OmpC and anti-I2 is plotted on the *y*-axis, and ANCA level is plotted on the *z*-axis. Reproduced with permission from the American Gastroenterological Association (Landers CJ, Cohavy O, Misra R, et al. Selected loss of tolerance evidenced by Crohn's disease-associated immune responses to auto- and microbial antigens. *Gastroenterology* 2002;123:689–99).

characteristics and genetic profiles of the populations, the correlations of response should be so close.

Conclusion

CD has many clinical manifestations, the impact of which on any individual is also influenced by environmental and psychological factors. There have been many attempts to classify these manifestations from a clinical and biological perspective. The potential advantages of accurate classification include the identification of subgroups that respond to specific treatments better than others, clarification of pathogenic mechanisms, and, more recently, relating genotype to phenotype. The identification of the potential pathogenic importance of the Paneth cell [43,44] is an example of how phenotypic associations have led to clarifications of the mechanisms of disease.

Clinical classifications of disease have received much attention and, although early classifications were difficult to calculate and reproduce, the Vienna classification has improved on many of these aspects. Classification of disease based on three variables (age at diagnosis, location of disease, and disease behavior) has led to an easily used and more reproducible index [16]. A number of difficulties remain with the Vienna classification. Although age at diagnosis does not change over the course of the disease, disease location and especially disease behavior are dynamic [18] and change significantly over the disease course. Change in disease location is relatively slow – it was only significant at 10 years following diagnosis in the analysis of Louis et al. [18] – and thus the Vienna definition of maximal extent prior to the first surgery removes this problem. This is not the case for disease behavior – indeed, it has been demonstrated that in excess of 80% of disease behaviors will change [14,18], and it may be more appropriate to classify the nature or even the speed of change, rather than to characterize this dynamic process at a single time point. The relevance of these changes is demonstrated by the protective role of NOD2/CARD15 in the development of penetrating disease.

A further difficulty with the Vienna classification is the inclusion of perianal disease as penetrating disease. Our own group and others have demonstrated that the presence of perianal penetrating disease is independent of internal penetrating disease [90], carrying different consequences in terms of the need for surgery. It is also argued that inclusion of perianal disease as penetrating disease, together with the hierarchical nature of the classification, may miss the primary disease phenotype. There is now a coherent argument in favor of classifying perianal disease as a separate category or subcategory within the Vienna classification. However, with each alteration or additional category, the classifications will tend to become more cumbersome and difficult to use.

More recent attempts to classify CD have been catalyzed by progress in our understanding of the molecular genetics of the disease and the need to relate genotype to disease phenotype. Indeed, it is increasingly clear that while assigning disease phenotype may be difficult, it is critical in determining the successful outcome of genetic association and linkage studies. The Toronto group has estimated that the erroneous assignation of phenotype may lead to a 40% loss of power in linkage studies [40]. Nonetheless, significant progress has been made in understanding CD genetics, illustrated most effectively by the identification of *NOD2/CARD15* as the *IBD1* gene.

The contribution of *NOD2/CARD15* to CD varies between populations, which is illustrated by the population attributable risk percentage. This is an estimate of the proportion of the disease in a population that can be attributed to the particular mutation. The population attributable risk percentage in data sets from Los Angeles [26] and the UK [29] was 27%. This compares with 33% in the initial French study of Hugot et al. [25], but only 12.9% in a Finnish cohort [38], 11% in our Scottish cohort [91], and 0% in a small Icelandic cohort [39]. It is therefore clear that there are many other genetic determinants to be characterized in CD.

Serological markers of IBD have been assessed since the 1950s, with the first report of ASCA in CD published from a Scottish population in 1988 [92]. It has subsequently transpired that, even with a combination of markers, these tests lack the sensitivity and specificity to be used as screening tools for IBD [73]. Use has been demonstrated in the stratification of disease, differentiating

CD from UC, and accelerating a diagnosis in patients with indeterminate colitis. Despite these data, serological markers have not been widely used in European populations, but are used considerably more often in North America. In addition, there have been variable reports of the association of serology with phenotype of disease, but emerging data are suggesting that cumulative presence and magnitude of response to a number of microbial antigens may be a sensitive marker of severe disease characterized by small bowel disease, frequent surgery, penetrating disease, and progression of disease type. These markers, although possibly acquired over the course of the disease, are stable over short periods of time and may yet prove to be useful disease markers.

Previous data have demonstrated links between serology and genetic markers in both CD and UC [93]. The emergence of these novel phenotypic associations with newer serological markers identifies the need to re-examine serotype–genotype associations further. It remains clear, however, that the most useful aspects of subclinical markers have yet to be realized. Although pANCA has been shown to identify patients at high risk for pouchitis prior to forthcoming pouch surgery [94], few data exist regarding the use of pANCA in determining treatment response, need for surgery, disease behavior, or short- to long-term prognosis. It is in this area that tangible benefits to patients should be sought and may yet be seen.

References

1. Crohn BB, Ginzburg L, Oppenheimer GD. Regional ileitis. A pathological and clinical entity. *JAMA* 1932;99:1323–9.
2. Bouma G, Strober W. The immunological and genetic basis of inflammatory bowel disease. *Nat Rev Immunol* 2003;3:521–33.
3. Lennard-Jones JE. Classification of inflammatory bowel disease. *Scand J Gastroenterol Suppl* 1989;170:2–6; discussion 16–19.
4. Farmer RG, Hawk WA, Turnbull RB Jr. Clinical patterns in Crohn's disease: a statistical study of 615 cases. *Gastroenterology* 1975;68:627–35.
5. Farmer RG, Whelan G, Fazio VW. Long-term follow-up of patients with Crohn's disease. Relationship between the clinical pattern and prognosis. *Gastroenterology* 1985;88:1818–25.

6. Gross V, Andus T, Caesar I, et al. Oral pH-modified release budesonide versus 6-methylprednisolone in active Crohn's disease. German/Austrian Budesonide Study Group. *Eur J Gastroenterol Hepatol* 1996;8:905–9.

7. Griffiths AM, Wesson DE, Shandling B, et al. Factors influencing postoperative recurrence of Crohn's disease in childhood. *Gut* 1991;32:491–5.

8. Greenstein AJ, Lachman P, Sachar DB, et al. Perforating and non-perforating indications for repeated operations in Crohn's disease: evidence for two clinical forms. *Gut* 1988;29:588–92.

9. Sachar DB, Andrews HA, Farmer RG, et al. Proposed classification of patient subgroups in Crohn's disease. *Gastroenterol Intl* 1992;5:141–54.

10. Steinhart AH, Girgrah N, McLeod RS. Reliability of a Crohn's disease clinical classification scheme based on disease behavior. *Inflamm Bowel Dis* 1998;4:228–34.

11. Aeberhard P, Berchtold W, Riedtmann HJ, et al. Surgical recurrence of perforating and nonperforating Crohn's disease. A study of 101 surgically treated patients. *Dis Colon Rectum* 1996;39:80–7.

12. Smith BKR, Arnott ID, Drummond HE, et al. Disease location, anti-*Saccharomyces cerevisiae* antibody (ASCA) and NOD2/CARD15 genotype influence the progression of disease behaviour in Crohn's disease. *Inflamm Bowel Dis* 2004 (In press).

13. Hamon JF, Carbonnel F, Beaugerie L, et al. Comparison of long-term course of perforating and non-perforating Crohn disease. *Gastroenterol Clin Biol* 1998;22:601–6 (In French).

14. Cosnes J, Cattan S, Blain A, et al. Long-term evolution of disease behavior of Crohn's disease. *Inflamm Bowel Dis* 2002;8:244–50.

15. Gasche C, Scholmerich J, Brynskov J, et al. A simple classification of Crohn's disease: report of the Working Party for the World Congresses of Gastroenterology, Vienna 1998. *Inflamm Bowel Dis* 2000;6:8–15.

16. Achkar JP, Brzezinski A. Interobserver agreement for disease behaviour phenotype in Crohn's disease. *Gastroenterology* 2002;122:W1293 (Abstr.).

17. Murillo L, Crusius JB, van Bodegraven AA, et al. CARD15 gene and the classification of Crohn's disease. *Immunogenetics* 2002;54:59–61.

18. Louis E, Collard A, Oger AF, et al. Behaviour of Crohn's disease according to the Vienna classification: changing pattern over the course of the disease. *Gut* 2001;49:777–82.

19. Louis E, Michel V, Hugot JP, et al. Early development of stricturing or penetrating pattern in Crohn's disease is influenced by disease location, number of flares, and smoking but not by *NOD2/CARD15* genotype. *Gut* 2003;52:552–7.

20. Rioux JD, Daly MJ, Silverberg MS, et al. Genetic variation in the 5q31 cytokine gene cluster confers susceptibility to Crohn disease. *Nat Genet* 2001;29:223–8.

21. Russell RK, Satsangi J. IBD: a family affair. *Best Pract Res Clin Gastroenterol* 2004;18:525–39.

22. Polito JM, Childs B, Mellits ED, et al. Crohn's disease: influence of age at diagnosis on site and clinical type of disease. *Gastroenterology* 1996;111:580–6.

23. Satsangi J, Morecroft J, Shah NB, et al. Genetics of inflammatory bowel disease: scientific and clinical implications. *Best Pract Res Clin Gastroenterol* 2003;17:3–18.

24. Ogura Y, Bonen DK, Inohara N, et al. A frameshift mutation in NOD2 associated with susceptibility to Crohn's disease. *Nature* 2001;411:603–6.

25. Hugot JP, Chamaillard M, Zouali H, et al. Association of NOD2 leucine-rich repeat variants with susceptibility to Crohn's disease. *Nature* 2001;411:599–603.

26. Abreu MT, Taylor KD, Lin YC, et al. Mutations in NOD2 are associated with fibrostenosing disease in patients with Crohn's disease. *Gastroenterology* 2002;123:679–88.

27. Vermeire S, Wild G, Kocher K, et al. CARD15 genetic variation in a Quebec population: prevalence, genotype–phenotype relationship, and haplotype structure. *Am J Hum Genet* 2002;71:74–83.
28. Cuthbert AP, Fisher SA, Mirza MM, et al. The contribution of NOD2 gene mutations to the risk and site of disease in inflammatory bowel disease. *Gastroenterology* 2002;122:867–74.
29. Ahmad T, Armuzzi A, Bunce M, et al. The molecular classification of the clinical manifestations of Crohn's disease. *Gastroenterology* 2002;122:854–66.
30. Lesage S, Zouali H, Cezard JP, et al. CARD15/NOD2 mutational analysis and genotype–phenotype correlation in 612 patients with inflammatory bowel disease. *Am J Hum Genet* 2002;70:845–57.
31. Yamazaki K, Takazoe M, Tanaka T, et al. Absence of mutation in the NOD2/CARD15 gene among 483 Japanese patients with Crohn's disease. *J Hum Genet* 2002;47:469–72.
32. Inoue N, Tamura K, Kinouchi Y, et al. Lack of common NOD2 variants in Japanese patients with Crohn's disease. *Gastroenterology* 2002;123:86–91.
33. Croucher PJ, Mascheretti S, Hampe J, et al. Haplotype structure and association to Crohn's disease of CARD15 mutations in two ethnically divergent populations. *Eur J Hum Genet* 2003;11:6–16.
34. Bonen DK, Ogura Y, Nicolae DL, et al. Crohn's disease-associated NOD2 variants share a signaling defect in response to lipopolysaccharide and peptidoglycan. *Gastroenterology* 2003;124:140–6.
35. Sugimura K, Taylor KD, Lin YC, et al. A novel NOD2/CARD15 haplotype conferring risk for Crohn disease in Ashkenazi Jews. *Am J Hum Genet* 2003;72:509–18.
36. Bairead E, Harmon DL, Curtis AM, et al. Association of NOD2 with Crohn's disease in a homogenous Irish population. *Eur J Hum Genet* 2003;11:237–44.
37. Hampe J, Grebe J, Nikolaus S, et al. Association of NOD2 (CARD 15) genotype with clinical course of Crohn's disease: a cohort study. *Lancet* 2002;359:1661–5.
38. Helio T, Halme L, Lappalainen M, et al. CARD15/NOD2 gene variants are associated with familially occurring and complicated forms of Crohn's disease. *Gut* 2003;52:558–62.
39. Thjodleifsson B, Sigthorsson G, Cariglia N, et al. Subclinical intestinal inflammation: an inherited abnormality in Crohn's disease relatives? *Gastroenterology* 2003;124:1728–37.
40. Silverberg MS, Daly MJ, Moskovitz DN, et al. Diagnostic misclassification reduces the ability to detect linkage in inflammatory bowel disease genetic studies. *Gut* 2001;49:773–6.
41. Tomer G, Ceballos C, Concepcion E, et al. NOD2/CARD15 variants are associated with lower weight at diagnosis in children with Crohn's disease. *Am J Gastroenterol* 2003;98:2479–84.
42. Brant SR, Picco MF, Achkar JP, et al. Defining complex contributions of NOD2/CARD15 gene mutations, age at onset, and tobacco use on Crohn's disease phenotypes. *Inflamm Bowel Dis* 2003;9:281–9.
43. Ogura Y, Lala S, Xin W, et al. Expression of NOD2 in Paneth cells: a possible link to Crohn's ileitis. *Gut* 2003;52:1591–7.
44. Lala S, Ogura Y, Osborne C, et al. Crohn's disease and the NOD2 gene: a role for Paneth cells. *Gastroenterology* 2003;125:47–57.
45. Hampe J, Cuthbert A, Croucher PJ, et al. Association between insertion mutation in NOD2 gene and Crohn's disease in German and British populations. *Lancet* 2001;357:1925–8.

46. Radlmayr M, Torok HP, Martin K, et al. The c-insertion mutation of the NOD2 gene is associated with fistulizing and fibrostenotic phenotypes in Crohn's disease. *Gastroenterology* 2002;122:2091–2.

47. Arnott ID, Satsangi J. Crohn's disease or Crohn's diseases? *Gut* 2003;52:460–1.

48. Satsangi J, Welsh KI, Bunce M, et al. Contribution of genes of the major histocompatibility complex to susceptibility and disease phenotype in inflammatory bowel disease. *Lancet* 1996;347:1212–17.

49. Hampe J, Shaw SH, Saiz R, et al. Linkage of inflammatory bowel disease to human chromosome 6p. *Am J Hum Genet* 1999;6:1647–55.

50. van Heel DA, Dechairo BM, Dawson G, et al. The IBD6 Crohn's disease locus demonstrates complex interactions with CARD15 and IBD5 disease-associated variants. *Hum Mol Genet* 2003;12:2569–75.

51. Nakajima A, Matsuhashi N, Kodama T, et al. HLA-linked susceptibility and resistance genes in Crohn's disease. *Gastroenterology* 1995;109:1462–7.

52. Stokkers PC, Reitsma PH, Tytgat GN, et al. HLA-DR and -DQ phenotypes in inflammatory bowel disease: a meta-analysis. *Gut* 1999;45:395–401.

53. Hesresbach D, Alizadeh M, Bretagne JF, et al. Investigation of the association of major histocompatibility complex genes, including HLA class I, class II and TAP genes, with clinical forms of Crohn's disease. *Eur J Immunogenet* 1996;23:141–51.

54. Kinouchi Y, Matsumoto K, Negoro K, et al. HLA-B genotype in Japanese patients with Crohn's disease. *Dis Colon Rectum* 2003;46(10 Suppl.):S10–4.

55. Orchard TR, Thiyagaraja S, Welsh KI, et al. Clinical phenotype is related to HLA genotype in the peripheral arthropathies of inflammatory bowel disease. *Gastroenterology* 2000;118:274–8.

56. Bonen DK, Cho JH. The genetics of inflammatory bowel disease. *Gastroenterology* 2003;124:521–36.

57. Roussomoustakaki M, Satsangi J, Welsh K, et al. Genetic markers may predict disease behavior in patients with ulcerative colitis. *Gastroenterology* 1997;112:1845–53.

58. Trachtenberg EA, Yang H, Hayes E, et al. HLA class II haplotype associations with inflammatory bowel disease in Jewish (Ashkenazi) and non-Jewish Caucasian populations. *Hum Immunol* 2000;61:326–33.

59. Futami S, Aoyama N, Honsako Y, et al. HLA-DRB1*1502 allele, subtype of DR15, is associated with susceptibility to ulcerative colitis and its progression. *Dig Dis Sci* 1995;40:814–18.

60. Rioux JD, Silverberg MS, Daly MJ, et al. Genome-wide search in Canadian families with inflammatory bowel disease reveals two novel susceptibility loci. *Am J Hum Genet* 2000;66:1863–70.

61. Mirza MM, Fisher SA, King K, et al. Genetic evidence for interaction of the 5q31 cytokine locus and the CARD15 gene in Crohn disease. *Am J Hum Genet* 2003;72:1018–22.

62. Giallourakis C, Stoll M, Miller K, et al. IBD5 is a general risk factor for inflammatory bowel disease: replication of association with Crohn disease and identification of a novel association with ulcerative colitis. *Am J Hum Genet* 2003;73:205–11.

63. Armuzzi A, Ahmad T, Ling KL, et al. Genotype–phenotype analysis of the Crohn's disease susceptibility haplotype on chromosome 5q31. *Gut* 2003;52:1133–9.

64. Kuhn R, Lohler J, Rennick D, et al. Interleukin-10-deficient mice develop chronic enterocolitis. *Cell* 1993;75:263–74.

65. D'Haens GR, Geboes K, Peeters M, et al. Early lesions of recurrent Crohn's disease caused by infusion of intestinal contents in excluded ileum. *Gastroenterology* 1998;114:262–7.

66. Turunen UM, Farkkila MA, Hakala K, et al. Long-term treatment of ulcerative colitis with ciprofloxacin: a prospective, double-blind, placebo-controlled study. *Gastroenterology* 1998;115:1072–8.

67. Arnold GL, Beaves MR, Pryjdun VO, et al. Preliminary study of ciprofloxacin in active Crohn's disease. *Inflamm Bowel Dis* 2002;8:10–15.

68. Gionchetti P, Rizzello F, Helwig U, et al. Prophylaxis of pouchitis onset with probiotic therapy: a double-blind, placebo-controlled trial. *Gastroenterology* 2003;124:1202–9.

69. Girardin SE, Boneca IG, Viala J, et al. Nod2 is a general sensor of peptidoglycan through muramyl dipeptide (MDP) detection. *J Biol Chem* 2003;278:8869–72.

70. Mahler M, Leiter EH. Genetic and environmental context determines the course of colitis developing in IL-10-deficient mice. *Inflamm Bowel Dis* 2002;8:347–55.

71. Landers CJ, Cohavy O, Misra R, et al. Selected loss of tolerance evidenced by Crohn's disease-associated immune responses to auto- and microbial antigens. *Gastroenterology* 2002;123:689–99.

72. Duchmann R, May E, Heike M, et al. T cell specificity and cross reactivity towards enterobacteria, bacteroides, bifidobacterium, and antigens from resident intestinal flora in humans. *Gut* 1999;44:812–18.

73. Reumaux D, Sendid B, Poulain D, et al. Serological markers in inflammatory bowel diseases. *Best Pract Res Clin Gastroenterol* 2003;17:19–35.

74. Koutroubakis IE, Petinaki E, Mouzas IA, et al. Anti-*Saccharomyces cerevisiae* mannan antibodies and antineutrophil cytoplasmic autoantibodies in Greek patients with inflammatory bowel disease. *Am J Gastroenterol* 2001;96:449–54.

75. Quinton JF, Sendid B, Reumaux D, et al. Anti-*Saccharomyces cerevisiae* mannan antibodies combined with antineutrophil cytoplasmic autoantibodies in inflammatory bowel disease: prevalence and diagnostic role. *Gut* 1998;42:788–91.

76. Hertervig E, Wieslander J, Johansson C, et al. Anti-neutrophil cytoplasmic antibodies in chronic inflammatory bowel disease. Prevalence and diagnostic role. *Scand J Gastroenterol* 1995;30:693–8.

77. Seibold F, Weber P, Schoning A, et al. Neutrophil antibodies (pANCA) in chronic liver disease and inflammatory bowel disease: do they react with different antigens? *Eur J Gastroenterol Hepatol* 1996;8:1095–100.

78. Abad E, Tural C, Mirapeix E, et al. Relationship between ANCA and clinical activity in inflammatory bowel disease: variation in prevalence of ANCA and evidence of heterogeneity. *J Autoimmun* 1997;10:175–80.

79. Duerr RH, Targan SR, Landers CJ, et al. Anti-neutrophil cytoplasmic antibodies in ulcerative colitis. Comparison with other colitides/diarrheal illnesses. *Gastroenterology* 1991;100:1590–6.

80. Freeman HJ. Inflammatory bowel disease with cytoplasmic-staining antineutrophil cytoplasmic antibody and extensive colitis. *Can J Gastroenterol* 1998;12:279–82.

81. Vasiliauskas EA, Kam LY, Karp LC, et al. Marker antibody expression stratifies Crohn's disease into immunologically homogeneous subgroups with distinct clinical characteristics. *Gut* 2000;47:487–96.

82. Vermeire S, Peeters M, Vlietinck R, et al. Anti-*Saccharomyces cerevisiae* antibodies (ASCA), phenotypes of IBD, and intestinal permeability: a study in IBD families. *Inflamm Bowel Dis* 2001;7:8–15.

83. Joossens S, Vermeire S, Claessens G, et al. Stratification of Crohn's disease (CD) patients according to their ASCA (anti-*Saccharomyces cerevisiae* antibodies) expression. *Gastroenterology* 2003;122:A266 (Abstr.).

84. Vasiliauskas EA, Plevy SE, Landers CJ, et al. Perinuclear antineutrophil cytoplasmic antibodies in patients with Crohn's disease define a clinical subgroup. *Gastroenterology* 1996;110:1810–19.

85. Jamar-Leclerc N, Reumaux D, Duthilleul P, et al. Do pANCA define a clinical subgroup in patients with Crohn's disease? *Gastroenterology* 1997;112:316–17.

86. Klebl FH, Bataille F, Bertea CR, et al. Association of perinuclear antineutrophil cytoplasmic antibodies and anti-*Saccharomyces cerevisiae* antibodies with Vienna classification subtypes of Crohn's disease. *Inflamm Bowel Dis* 2003;9:302–7.

87. Sendid B, Quinton JF, Charrier G, et al. Anti-*Saccharomyces cerevisiae* mannan antibodies in familial Crohn's disease. *Am J Gastroenterol* 1998;93:1306–10.

88. Sutton CL, Yang H, Li Z, et al. Familial expression of anti-*Saccharomyces cerevisiae* mannan antibodies in affected and unaffected relatives of patients with Crohn's disease. *Gut* 2000;46:58–63.

89. Mow WS, Vasiliauskas EA, Lin YC, et al. Association of antibody reponses to microbial antigens and complications of small bowel Crohn's disease. *Gastroenterology* 2004;126:414–24.

90. Veloso FT, Ferreira JT, Barros L, et al. Clinical outcome of Crohn's disease: analysis according to the Vienna classification and clinical activity. *Inflamm Bowel Dis* 2001;7:306–13.

91. Arnott IDR, Nimmo ER, Drummond HE, et al. *NOD2*, *CARD15*, *TLR4* and *CD14* mutations in Scottish and Irish Crohn's disease patients: evidence for genetic heterogeneity within Euorpe? *Genes Immun* 2004 (In press).

92. Main J, McKenzie H, Yeaman GR, et al. Antibody to *Saccharomyces cerevisiae* (bakers' yeast) in Crohn's disease. *Br Med J* 1988;297:1105–6.

93. Satsangi J, Landers CJ, Welsh KI, et al. The presence of anti-neutrophil antibodies reflects clinical and genetic heterogeneity within inflammatory bowel disease. *Inflamm Bowel Dis* 1998;4:18–26.

94. Fleshner PR, Vasiliauskas EA, Kam LY, et al. High level perinuclear antineutrophil cytoplasmic antibody (pANCA) in ulcerative colitis patients before colectomy predicts the development of chronic pouchitis after ileal pouch-anal anastomosis. *Gut* 2001;49:671–7.

95. Bernstein CN, Orr K, Blanchard JF, et al. Development of an assay for antibodies to *Saccharomyces cerevisiae*: Easy, cheap and specific for Crohn's disease. *Can J Gastroenterol* 2001;15:499–504.

96. Peeters M, Joossens S, Vermeire S, et al. Diagnostic value of anti-*Saccharomyces cerevisiae* and antineutrophil cytoplasmic autoantibodies in inflammatory bowel disease. *Am J Gastroenterol* 2001;96:730–4.

3

Nutrition therapy

Donald R Duerksen

Introduction

Malnutrition is a common and significant complication of ulcerative colitis (UC) and Crohn's disease (CD). In the past decade there have been significant advances in nutritional therapies, particularly in the use of specialized nutrients such as omega-3 fatty acids, glutamine, short-chain fatty acids, and folic acid. In addition, numerous randomized controlled studies have examined the role of nutrition therapy in inflammatory bowel disease.

A major difference between UC and CD is the significant effect that nutrition, in particular enteral nutrition, can have on the treatment of active disease. In this chapter, we consider the prevalence of malnutrition in UC and CD and discuss the role of enteral nutrition, total parenteral nutrition (TPN), and specialized nutrients in the management of these disorders.

Crohn's disease

Protein calorie malnutrition

Malnutrition is very common in CD, with an incidence ranging from 25% to 80% [1]. The best method for detecting protein calorie malnutrition in CD is unclear. Subjective global assessment (see **Table 1**) [2] has been validated in other patient populations and its general applicability suggests that it is also likely to be valid in CD, although it has not been specifically

A. History	
1. Weight change	Overall weight loss in past 6 months: __ kg __ %
	Change in past 2 weeks: __ increase __ no change __ decrease
2. Dietary intake change (relative to normal)	No change Change: __ duration = #__ weeks Type: __ suboptimal solid diet __ hypocaloric liquids __ full liquid diet __ starvation
3. Gastrointestinal symptoms (that persisted for >2 weeks)	__ none __ nausea __ vomiting __ diarrhea
4. Functional capacity	__ no dysfunction (eg, full capacity) __ dysfunction __ duration = #__ weeks Type: __ working suboptimally __ ambulatory __ bedridden
5. Disease and its relation to nutritional requirements	Primary diagnosis (specify) _____ Metabolic demand (stress): __ no stress __ low stress __ moderate stress __ high stress

Table 1. Subjective global assessment (SGA). Adapted with permission from the American Society for Parenteral & Enteral Nutrition (Detsky AS, McLaughlin JR, Baker JP, et al. What is the subjective global assessment of nutritional status? *JPEN J Parenter Enteral Nutr* 1987;11:8–13).

B. Physical

(For each trait specify: 0 = normal, 1+ = mild or moderate, 2+ = severe)

__ loss of subcutaneous fat (triceps, chest)

__ muscle wasting (quadriceps, deltoids)

__ edema

__ sacral edema

__ ascites

SGA rating (select one)

__ A = well nourished

__ B = moderately malnourished

__ C = severely malnourished

Table 1. *Continued.*

tested in this area [1]. Hypoalbuminemia is a frequent finding in active CD [3], but is more likely to be related to disease activity than to malnutrition [4]. Decreased oral intake is the primary cause of malnutrition [5], although several other factors may also contribute, including malabsorption [3] and increased resting energy expenditure in septic or underweight patients [6,7].

Enteral nutrition is the treatment of choice based on its ability to improve body composition and promote weight gain, even in patients with active CD [8]. In the out-patient management of CD patients, nutritional supplements should be instituted in nutritionally at-risk patients. The timing of specific nutritional intervention and the effect of nutritional support on clinically based outcomes such as infectious complications and functional status have not been well defined in CD.

Micronutrient deficiencies

In addition to protein calorie malnutrition, patients with CD are at risk for developing vitamin and other micronutrient deficiencies. The following micronutrient deficiencies have been described: vitamins A, D, and E, thiamine, riboflavin, folate, vitamin B_{12}, iron, calcium, magnesium, potassium, selenium, and

Deficiency	Prevalence
Iron	39
Folate	54
Vitamin B_{12}	48
Calcium	13
Magnesium	14–88
Potassium	6–20
Zinc	40–50
Vitamin A	11
Vitamin D	75
Selenium	35–40

Table 2. Vitamin, mineral and trace element deficiencies in Crohn's disease. (Data from Dieleman LA, Heizer WD. Nutritional issues in inflammatory bowel disease. *Gastroenterol Clin North Am* 1998;27:435–51 and Kelly DG, Fleming CR. Nutritional consideration in inflammatory bowel diseases. *Gastroenterol Clin North Am* 1995;24:597–611.)

zinc (see **Table 2**) [3]. The etiology of these deficiencies relates to several factors, including decreased oral intake, increased losses (due to underlying diarrhea), and malabsorption (eg, of vitamin B_{12} in patients with ileal disease or resection). The clinical effects of these deficiencies may often be unnoticeable in CD patients and a high index of suspicion is required. Given the high prevalence of deficiencies, we would recommend that all patients be given a multivitamin/mineral supplement.

CD patients have an increased incidence of osteoporosis [9] and a higher fracture rate compared with the general population [10], and all patients should be assessed to ensure that their calcium (1,000 mg/day elemental calcium for individuals <50 years old; 1,500 mg/day for those >50 years old) and vitamin D (400–800 IU/day) intakes are optimized. Milk and milk products are the best dietary source of calcium. While there is an increased prevalence of lactase deficiency in CD [11], but not in UC [12], many CD patients tolerate up to 250 mL of milk per day [13].

Enteral feeding for the treatment of active CD

In 1973, Voitk et al. noted that patients who received nutritional therapy prior to surgery frequently went into clinical remission [14]. This led to the hypothesis that enteral feeding may have a primary role in the treatment of active CD. Subsequently, many small prospective studies have examined the effect of enteral feeding on CD (although there have been no large randomized placebo-controlled studies on the subject). Most studies have compared enteral feeding with corticosteroids, which induce a remission rate of ~80% [15].

Early trials examining the role of enteral nutrition in active CD demonstrated a 60%–80% remission rate [16–18]. Three meta-analyses in the mid 1990s examined trials of enteral feeding in CD. They concluded that enteral feeding is not as effective as corticosteroid therapy, but that remission rates are approximately 60%, which is considerably greater than the placebo response of 20% found in drug trials for CD [19–21]. More recently, a systematic review of studies examining the role of enteral feeding in active CD by the Cochrane collaboration has come to similar conclusions [22]. The response rates may be different in pediatric populations, where a meta-analysis showed equivalent response to steroids and improved growth in enterally fed individuals [23].

Mechanism

The mechanism by which enteral nutrition induces clinical remission in CD remains unclear [1]. Hypotheses include:

- reduced antigenicity of the luminal contents due to the absence of whole protein

- exclusion of dietary components not found in enteral formula diets

- alteration of host bacterial flora

- reduction of total fat

- alteration of fatty acid content, resulting in a reduction of inflammation by decreasing eicosanoid precursors

- decreasing colonic fecal bile salt load (due to low-fat diets decreasing enterohepatic circulation of bile acids)

- the provision of specialized nutrients such as glutamine in chemically defined diets

Bowel rest does not appear to be of major importance in effecting a remission [24].

One recent theory regarding the role of diet in activating CD suggests that microparticles may play a part [25]. This hypothesis states that microparticles such as titanium dioxide and aluminosilicates may adsorb luminal constituents and activate intestinal phagocytes. A clinical study that randomized 20 patients to either a control diet or a low-microparticle diet demonstrated a significantly reduced Crohn's disease activity index (CDAI) in the low-microparticle group [26]. This theory requires further study and validation.

The mechanism by which enteral nutrition benefits patients has practical relevance in that different compositions of enteral formulas may have different clinical effects. The most effective type of enteral formula is controversial, with most randomized controlled studies demonstrating no significant difference between elemental and polymeric formulas [27–29]. Therefore, it is unlikely that protein antigenicity accounts for the benefits of enteral feeding. No definitive conclusions were drawn regarding the type of formula from the meta-analyses of the Cochrane collaboration because of the small number of patients studied [20–22,30].

The role of fat
There has been much recent interest regarding the amount and type of fat ingested and the effect on CD activity. Over 90% of

dietary fat consists of triglycerides, which are structurally composed of a glycerol backbone and three fatty acids. Fatty acids are subclassified according to:

- the number of carbons (short-chain fatty acids have 2–6 carbons; medium-chain fatty acids have 8–12 carbons; long-chain fatty acids have 14–22 carbons)

- the presence or absence of double bonds (unsaturated or saturated, respectively)

Unsaturated fatty acids are further subclassified into omega-3 or omega-6 series, depending on the location of the first double bond.

Linoleic acid (C18:2ω6) is one of two essential fatty acids. It is the precursor to arachidonic acid, which is subsequently metabolized into 4-series leukotrienes and 2-series prostaglandins. These are proinflammatory cytokines, and could potentially worsen inflammatory states. Conversely, omega-3 fatty acids (commonly found in fish oils) may have an anti-inflammatory effect because of the types of leukotrienes (5-series) and prostaglandins (3-series) produced from the omega-3 series. Omega-3 and omega-6 fatty acids compete for desaturase and elongase enzymes, which metabolize long-chain fatty acids; therefore, provision of one source will alter production of the other.

Support for the role of fat in CD comes from both epidemiologic and basic science studies. In Japan, increased consumption of animal fat and omega-6 fatty acid composition in recent years may be responsible for the rising incidence of CD in the population [31]. Patients with longstanding CD have a lower omega-3 fatty acid composition of their plasma phospholipid and adipose stores compared with controls [32]. A meta-analysis of enteral feeding trials demonstrated decreased effectiveness of enteral formulas with increasing amounts of long-chain triglycerides [33].

Studies examining the role of fat content and composition in inducing remission in CD have yielded conflicting results. In a study of 36 patients with active CD who were randomized to receive one of three elemental formulas (3 g/day, 16 g/day, or 30 g/day of fat), the remission rates were significantly different at 4 weeks (80%, 40%, and 25%, respectively) [34]. The added fat was predominantly long-chain triglycerides, with 51.6% linoleic acid and 23.9% oleic acid. Therefore, this study supports the hypothesis that a high amount of fat (and particularly long-chain triglycerides in the form of linoleic and oleic acid) may result in lower remission rates.

Gassull et al. demonstrated that a polymeric formula high in linoleic acid (45%) and low in oleic acid (28.2%) was significantly more efficacious in inducing remission than a diet low in linoleic acid (6.5%) and high in oleic acid (79%) [35]. While this was a small study that randomized only 66 patients to one of three arms, the per protocol analysis demonstrated a significant benefit in terms of clinical remission in the high linoleic acid group (27% vs 63%). This is a surprising finding, as the study hypothesis was that a diet high in linoleic acid could lead to the production of proinflammatory eicosanoids and cytokines. It may be that diets high in oleic acid are also potentially deleterious.

A third study compared two polymeric feeds that differed in the amount of long-chain triglycerides supplied: 30% vs 5% of total energy [36]. Both groups had a similar remission rate, but the overall remission rates were quite low (33% and 26%, respectively) and the validity of these results therefore needs to be questioned. Studies have shown no detrimental effect of medium-chain triglycerides on the ability of enteral feeding to induce a clinical remission [30,37]. Further studies on the optimal fat content of enteral formulas for patients with CD need to be performed. Until these are available and the role of fat in CD is clarified, formulas with minimal fat, and in particular low in long-chain triglycerides, are preferred [38].

There are few data as to whether particular subgroups of patients may respond to enteral feeding. There may be a subset of patients who benefit from enteral nutrition after failing steroid therapy [39].

Summary
Enteral nutrition has a response rate of approximately 60% in active CD. The mechanism of action is unknown, but may relate to fat content. Pediatric populations may benefit more than adults and have the added benefit of improved growth. Important clinical questions remain to be answered, including the use of enteral nutrition in steroid refractory cases, the mechanism of enteral nutrition-induced clinical remission, and the optimal formula for inducing remission in CD.

Enteral feeding for the maintenance of remission
Even fewer studies have examined the role of enteral feeding in the maintenance of remission in CD patients. Two different enteral feeding approaches have been used to prevent flares of CD. The first approach allows patients to eat normally and at regular intervals, and then institutes exclusively enteral feeding for a prolonged period. Study protocols have typically allowed 3 months of *ad lib* diet followed by 1 month of exclusively enteral feeding [40,41]. These small controlled studies (N=6, N=8) have demonstrated decreased CDAI, decreased steroid use, and improved growth in patients receiving intermittent exclusive enteral feeding for 1 year as compared with the year prior to enteral feeding.

The second (perhaps more practical) approach is to administer daily nutritional supplements to individuals who have sustained a remission with enteral feeding. Harries et al. performed a randomized crossover study in which enterally treated patients received an average of 550 calories/day of an oral polymeric formula [42]. Compared with those receiving no supplement, these patients demonstrated improved anthropometrics, serum proteins, and creatinine height index. A retrospective study in which pediatric patients continued supplemental nutrition (a semi-elemental formula via a nasogastric tube 4–5 times/week) after remission was achieved with enteral feeding found an improved 1-year remission rate (57%) compared with patients not taking the supplements (21%) [43].

In a randomized controlled study of 39 patients, those receiving 760 kcal/day of an oral semi-elemental supplement showed an improved 1-year remission rate compared with patients who were maintained on a normal unrestricted diet with no supplementation (48% vs 22%) [44]. The same investigators also demonstrated similar 1-year remission rates when supplementation with semi-elemental and polymeric formulas was compared [45].

In summary, studies examining the role of enteral feeding in maintaining CD remission are smaller and less well controlled than those assessing its role in inducing remission. The available studies suggest a benefit with either intermittent exclusive supplementation or continuous partial supplementation. Further comparative studies with medication therapies are needed to define the role of enteral nutrition in maintaining remission in CD.

Fistulizing and perianal disease

The role of nutritional therapy in complex fistulas and severe refractory perianal disease is uncertain. No controlled studies have examined the role of TPN or enteral nutrition in fistulizing disease [46], although reports have associated TPN and enteral feeding with the closure of fistulas [47]. The optimum delivery of nutrition has not been studied, and the roles of bowel rest and TPN in this manifestation of CD are unknown. For distal fistulas, enteral feeding with an elemental formula may be tried. If the fistulas are more proximal in the small bowel or refractory to medical therapy, bowel rest and support with TPN may be attempted.

Use of percutaneous gastrostomy tubes

There is some concern that insertion of a percutaneous endoscopic gastrostomy (PEG) tube in a CD patient may lead to the development of peristomal CD or the formation of peristomal fistulas. However, because of the unpalatability of many of the elemental formulas and the need for prolonged enteral nutritional support in many patients with CD, a PEG tube is frequently the best device with which to facilitate optimal delivery of the enteral formula.

There are no prospective randomized trials comparing gastrostomy tube placement in patients with CD with other methods of enteral feeding. Case series have reported a total of 67 patients with gastrostomy tube insertions [48–51]. These series have demonstrated that a percutaneously inserted tube is often successful in cases where a nasogastric tube is not tolerated. They have also documented decreased steroid dosing and improved growth with enteral feeding through a gastrostomy tube. No insertional difficulties have been encountered in these individuals. There have been no reports of peristomal fistulas, and prolonged gastrocutaneous fistula after removal was rare. Therefore, in situations where prolonged enteral feeding is anticipated and nasogastric feeding is not tolerated or desired, a PEG tube should be considered.

Specialized nutrients

Glutamine

Glutamine, a conditionally essential amino acid, is the preferred fuel of the small bowel and may also have a role in regulating intestinal permeability [52] – intestinal permeability defects may be important in the pathogenesis of CD [53]. Therefore, there may be a role for glutamine supplementation in the management of acute CD. However, a study that randomized CD patients with an intestinal permeability defect to either 21 g of supplemental oral glutamine or placebo for 4 weeks found no improvement in intestinal permeability, CDAI, or nutritional status in the glutamine group [54]. A further study that compared a glutamine-enriched enteral formula with a standard isonitrogenous formula found no difference in remission rate. Therefore, despite theoretical considerations regarding the use of glutamine in CD, there is no evidence to support a clinical benefit.

Omega-3 fatty acids

The use of omega-3 fatty acids has been advocated in a variety of chronic inflammatory diseases due to their anti-inflammatory effects through several potential mechanisms [55]:

- reduced production of leukotriene B_4 and thromboxane A_2

- inhibition of inflammatory cytokines, such as interleukin-1 and tumor necrosis factor

- scavenging of free radicals

Several small clinical studies have demonstrated a clinical benefit from omega-3 fatty acids in CD patients. Belluzzi et al. demonstrated that after 1 year of treatment with 2.7 g of enteric-coated omega-3 fatty acids, 59% of patients remained in remission compared with 26% of patients on placebo [55]. While this trial showed significant benefit, another European study did not demonstrate any benefit in an intention-to-treat analysis [56]. Side-effects associated with omega-3 fatty acid supplementation include an unpleasant taste, halitosis, diarrhea, and flatulence.

Antioxidants

Individuals with CD show evidence of increased oxidative stress and decreased antioxidant defense compared with controls [57,58]. In a randomized controlled study, Geerling et al. demonstrated the normalization of antioxidant levels in CD patients who ingested beta carotene, vitamin E, and selenium, and an improved antioxidant status of patients in clinical remission [59]. In a study of clinically stable patients who were supplemented with vitamins C and E, the plasma levels of these vitamins increased and the measured oxidative stress decreased

[60]. These results provide evidence that antioxidant supplements may be useful in the treatment of CD and in maintenance of remission. Further clinical trials are needed in this area.

Elimination diets

It has been suggested that certain dietary components may be responsible for exacerbating CD, and that enteral formulas are effective in inducing remission because they eliminate the offending food component. Food intolerances have been reported in approximately 50% of patients with CD [61,62]. Although several European studies have examined the role of elimination diets in maintaining remission in patients with treated CD, this role is controversial. In a UK study, patients randomized to an elimination diet with no prednisone showed a significantly lower relapse rate at 2 years (62%) than patients who were tapered off prednisone over a 12-week period and given advice on healthy eating (79%) [63]. However, in a blinded controlled study examining the reproducibility of symptoms in patients who were rechallenged with a food component they had previously been identified as being sensitive to, there was a low rate of confirmation (24%) [62]. Given the difficulty with such diets and the limited data to support their use, we would agree with Pearson et al. who suggest that, "Food sensitivity is of insufficient importance to warrant putting all patients through elimination diets" [62].

Ulcerative colitis

Prevalence of malnutrition

The prevalence of malnutrition in UC is generally less than in CD and has been estimated to be 18%–62% [64]. Similarly, micronutrient deficiencies appear to be less common than in CD, with iron deficiency most frequently reported [3]. A study has demonstrated that, compared with controls, the serum levels of certain nutrients (zinc, selenium, beta carotene, and magnesium) were lower in UC patients studied within 6 months of their diagnosis [65].

The role of bowel rest and TPN in severe UC

In the late 1970s, a theory developed that "bowel rest" might be beneficial in treating active UC. Theories promoting the value of bowel rest cited less mechanical trauma, decreased intestinal secretions, and decreased antigenic load. Two studies have compared corticosteroid treatment and TPN with corticosteroids and an *ad lib* diet in patients with severe acute UC [66,67]. Bowel rest was not associated with any clinical benefit in either of these studies, and the rates of colectomy were similar in each group. In addition, unlike in CD, nutritional support with either TPN or enteral nutrition does not appear to have a primary role in controlling the underlying colitis. In the first of the two studies described above, rates of colectomy in severe acute colitis were high despite therapy with TPN [66].

In patients who are malnourished and require nutritional support, enteral feeding should initially be tried. Enteral feeding is frequently tolerated in this group of patients and has been associated with fewer complications when compared with TPN [68]. For patients who are intolerant of enteral nutrition but require nutritional support, TPN should be instituted. There are no prospective randomized studies examining the role of preoperative TPN in UC patients requiring TPN. A Veterans Affairs Cooperative Study that examined the role of preoperative TPN included patients with inflammatory bowel disease. In this study, preoperative TPN was only beneficial in individuals who were severely malnourished prior to surgery [69]. Until prospective studies suggest other indications, we would suggest using preoperative nutritional support only in patients who are severely malnourished.

Specialized nutrients

Short-chain fatty acids

Short-chain fatty acids are produced by intestinal bacteria from the fermentation of nondigestible starch. Short-chain fatty acids (in particular, butyrate) exert many effects on the colonic epithelial cell, including enhancing sodium and water absorption, serving as a preferential fuel, and exerting trophic effects [70].

Several controlled studies have examined the role of short-chain fatty acid enemas in the treatment of left-sided UC [35,71–73]. These studies have shown little or no clinical benefit, and the clinical utility of these therapies therefore appears small.

Recent studies have examined the potential of diets high in fiber, as a substrate for the production of short-chain fatty acids, to control UC [74,75]. These studies have demonstrated that it is possible to increase fecal butyrate levels with high-fiber diets. *Plantago ovata* seeds are a form of fermentable fiber, which, when given orally, yield high fecal concentrations of butyrate and acetate [76]. An open-label randomized study examining the role of these seeds in maintaining remission in UC demonstrated equal efficacy with mesalazine [77]. These are preliminary studies only, and larger controlled trials are necessary to determine the clinical role of these therapies.

Omega-3 fatty acids

Increased levels of the proinflammatory cytokines prostaglandin E_2 and leukotriene B_4 have been found in patients with UC [78]. The rationale for the use of omega-3 fatty acids was discussed earlier, and relates to the production of cytokines with less proinflammatory activity. Randomized controlled studies have demonstrated that fish oil supplementation decreases the activity of mild to moderate UC [79] and has a steroid-sparing effect [78,80], but appears to be less effective than 2 g/day of sulfasalazine in acute UC [81] and does not have a role in maintaining remission [80]. While omega-3 fatty acids have a biologic effect in UC, there currently appears to be little clinical role for their use in these patients.

Folic acid

Interest in folic acid supplementation has been stimulated by evidence that folate may have a role in the prevention of colon cancer in patients with longstanding UC [82–84], and may have a further role in decreasing thromboembolic disease [85,86]. Currently, no published prospective controlled studies have looked at the effectiveness of folate supplementation in the prevention of colon cancer or thromboembolic disease in UC patients. These will be needed before routine folic acid supplementation can be recommended for individuals with UC.

Conclusion

Patients with inflammatory bowel disease have a high incidence of protein calorie malnutrition and micronutrient deficiency. In CD, enteral feeding has a primary role in treating active disease. The mechanism of benefit is unknown, but may relate to the type and amount of fat in the formula. The optimal formula for inducing remission in CD is also unknown, but there does not appear to be a significant difference between polymeric and elemental formulas.

In UC, enteral nutrition does not have a role in the primary treatment of active disease; however, preliminary data suggest that high-fiber diets may play a part, particularly in maintaining UC remission. The role of specific micronutrient supplementation in CD and UC requires more clinical study before clinical recommendations can be made.

References

1. Goh J, O'Morain CA. Review article: nutrition and adult inflammatory bowel disease. *Aliment Pharmacol Ther* 2003;17:307–20.
2. Detsky AS, McLaughlin JR, Baker JP, et al. What is subjective global assessment of nutritional status? *JPEN J Parenter Enteral Nutr* 1987;11:8–13.
3. Kelly DG, Fleming CR. Nutritional considerations in inflammatory bowel diseases. *Gastroenterol Clin North Am* 1995;24:597–611.
4. Klein S. The myth of serum albumin as a measure of nutritional status. *Gastroenterology* 1990;99:1845–6.
5. Rigaud D, Angel LA, Cerf M, et al. Mechanisms of decreased food intake during weight loss in adult Crohn's disease patients without obvious malabsorption. *Am J Clin Nutr* 1994;60:775–81.
6. Chan AT, Fleming CR, O'Fallon WM, et al. Estimated versus measured basal energy requirements in patients with Crohn's disease. *Gastroenterology* 1986;91:75–8.
7. Stokes MA, Hill GL. Total energy expenditure in patients with Crohn's disease: measurement by the combined body scan technique. *JPEN J Parenter Enteral Nutr* 1993;17:3–7.

8. Royall D, Greenberg GR, Allard JP, et al. Total enteral nutrition support improves body composition of patients with active Crohn's disease. *JPEN J Parenter Enteral Nutr* 1995;19:95–9.

9. Bernstein CN, Leslie WD, Leboff MS. AGA technical review on osteoporosis in gastrointestinal diseases. *Gastroenterology* 2003;124:795–841.

10. Bernstein CN, Blanchard JF, Leslie W, et al. The incidence of fracture among patients with inflammatory bowel disease. A population-based cohort study. *Ann Intern Med* 2000;133:795–9.

11. Mishkin B, Yalovsky M, Mishkin S. Increased prevalence of lactose malabsorption in Crohn's disease patients at low risk for lactose malabsorption based on ethnic origin. *Am J Gastroenterol* 1997;92:1148–53.

12. Bernstein CN, Ament M, Artinian L, et al. Milk tolerance in adults with ulcerative colitis. *Am J Gastroenterol* 1994;89:872–7.

13. Pironi L, Callegari C, Cornia GL, et al. Lactose malabsorption in adult patients with Crohn's disease. *Am J Gastroenterol* 1988;83:1267–71.

14. Voitk AJ, Echave V, Feller JH, et al. Experience with elemental diet in the treatment of inflammatory bowel disease. Is this primary therapy? *Arch Surg* 1973;107:329–33.

15. Summers RW, Switz DM, Sessions JT Jr, et al. National Cooperative Crohn's Disease Study: results of drug treatment. *Gastroenterology* 1979;77:847–69.

16. Gonzalez-Huix F, de Leon R, Fernandez-Banares F, et al. Polymeric enteral diets as primary treatment of active Crohn's disease: a prospective steroid controlled trial. *Gut* 1993;34:778–82.

17. Lochs H, Steinhardt HJ, Klaus-Wentz B, et al. Comparison of enteral nutrition and drug treatment in active Crohn's disease. Results of the European Cooperative Crohn's Disease Study. IV. *Gastroenterology* 1991;101:881–8.

18. O'Morain C, Segal AW, Levi AJ. Elemental diet as primary treatment of acute Crohn's disease: a controlled trial. *Br Med J (Clin Res Ed)* 1984;288:1859–62.

19. Griffiths AM, Ohlsson A, Sherman PM, et al. Meta-analysis of enteral nutrition as a primary treatment of active Crohn's disease. *Gastroenterology* 1995;108:1056–67.

20. Fernandez-Banares F, Cabre E, Esteve-Comas M, et al. How effective is enteral nutrition in inducing clinical remission in active Crohn's disease? A meta-analysis of the randomized clinical trials. *JPEN J Parenter Enteral Nutr* 1995;19:356–64.

21. Messori A, Trallori G, D'Albasio G, et al. Defined-formula diets versus steroids in the treatment of active Crohn's disease: a meta-analysis. *Scand J Gastroenterol* 1996;31:267–72.

22. Zachos M, Tondeur M, Griffiths AM. Enteral nutritional therapy for inducing remission of Crohn's disease. *Cochrane Database Syst Rev* 2001:CD000542.

23. Heuschkel RB, Menache CC, Megerian JT, et al. Enteral nutrition and corticosteroids in the treatment of acute Crohn's disease in children. *J Pediatr Gastroenterol Nutr* 2000;31:8–15.

24. Greenberg GR, Fleming CR, Jeejeebhoy KN, et al. Controlled trial of bowel rest and nutritional support in the management of Crohn's disease. *Gut* 1988;29:1309–15.

25. Mahmud N, Weir DG. The urban diet and Crohn's disease: is there a relationship? *Eur J Gastroenterol Hepatol* 2001;13:93–5.

26. Lomer MC, Harvey RS, Evans SM, et al. Efficacy and tolerability of a low microparticle diet in a double blind, randomized, pilot study in Crohn's disease. *Eur J Gastroenterol Hepatol* 2001;13:101–6.

27. Rigaud D, Cosnes J, Le Quintrec Y, et al. Controlled trial comparing two types of enteral nutrition in treatment of active Crohn's disease: elemental versus polymeric diet. *Gut* 1991;32:1492–7.

28. Mansfield JC, Giaffer MH, Holdsworth CD. Controlled trial of oligopeptide versus amino acid diet in treatment of active Crohn's disease. *Gut* 1995;36:60–6.
29. Royall D, Jeejeebhoy KN, Baker JP, et al. Comparison of amino acid v peptide based enteral diets in active Crohn's disease: clinical and nutritional outcome. *Gut* 1994;35:783–7.
30. Sakurai T, Matsui T, Yao T, et al. Short-term efficacy of enteral nutrition in the treatment of active Crohn's disease: a randomized, controlled trial comparing nutrient formulas. *JPEN J Parenter Enteral Nutr* 2002;26:98–103.
31. Shoda R, Matsueda K, Yamato S, et al. Epidemiologic analysis of Crohn disease in Japan: increased dietary intake of n-6 polyunsaturated fatty acids and animal protein relates to the increased incidence of Crohn disease in Japan. *Am J Clin Nutr* 1996;63:741–5.
32. Geerling BJ, Houwelingen AC, Badart-Smook A, et al. Fat intake and fatty acid profile in plasma phospholipids and adipose tissue in patients with Crohn's disease, compared with controls. *Am J Gastroenterol* 1999;94:410–17.
33. Middleton SJ, Rucker JT, Kirby GA. Long-chain triglycerides reduce the efficacy of enteral feeds in patients with active Crohn's disease. *Clin Nutr* 1995;14:229–36.
34. Bamba T, Shimoyama T, Sasaki M, et al. Dietary fat attenuates the benefits of an elemental diet in active Crohn's disease: a randomized, controlled trial. *Eur J Gastroenterol Hepatol* 2003;15:151–7.
35. Gassull MA, Fernandez-Banares F, Cabre E, et al. Fat composition may be a clue to explain the primary therapeutic effect of enteral nutrition in Crohn's disease: results of a double blind randomised multicentre European trial. *Gut* 2002;51:164–8.
36. Leiper K, Woolner J, Mullan MM, et al. A randomised controlled trial of high versus low long chain triglyceride whole protein feed in active Crohn's disease. *Gut* 2001;49:790–4.
37. Khoshoo V, Reifen R, Neuman MG, et al. Effect of low- and high-fat, peptide-based diets on body composition and disease activity in adolescents with active Crohn's disease. *JPEN J Parenter Enteral Nutr* 1996;20:401–5.
38. Gorard DA. Enteral nutrition in Crohn's disease: fat in the formula. *Eur J Gastroenterol Hepatol* 2003;15:115–18.
39. O'Brien CJ, Giaffer MH, Cann PA, et al. Elemental diet in steroid-dependent and steroid-refractory Crohn's disease. *Am J Gastroenterol* 1991;86:1614–18.
40. Belli DC, Seidman E, Bouthillier L, et al. Chronic intermittent elemental diet improves growth failure in children with Crohn's disease. *Gastroenterology* 1988;94:603–10.
41. Polk DB, Hattner JA, Kerner JA Jr. Improved growth and disease activity after intermittent administration of a defined formula diet in children with Crohn's disease. *JPEN J Parenter Enteral Nutr* 1992;16:499–504.
42. Harries AD, Jones LA, Danis V, et al. Controlled trial of supplemented oral nutrition in Crohn's disease. *Lancet* 1983;1:887–90.
43. Wilschanski M, Sherman P, Pencharz P, et al. Supplementary enteral nutrition maintains remission in paediatric Crohn's disease. *Gut* 1996;38:543–8.
44. Verma S, Kirkwood B, Brown S, et al. Oral nutritional supplementation is effective in the maintenance of remission in Crohn's disease. *Dig Liver Dis* 2000;32:769–74.
45. Verma S, Holdsworth CD, Giaffer MH. Does adjuvant nutritional support diminish steroid dependency in Crohn disease? *Scand J Gastroenterol* 2001;36:383–8.
46. Wu S, Craig RM. Intense nutritional support in inflammatory bowel disease. *Dig Dis Sci* 1995;40:843–52.
47. Rombeau JL, Rolandelli RH. Enteral and parenteral nutrition in patients with enteric fistulas and short bowel syndrome. *Surg Clin North Am* 1987;67:551–71.

48. Israel DM, Hassall E. Prolonged use of gastrostomy for enteral hyperalimentation in children with Crohn's disease. *Am J Gastroenterol* 1995;90:1084–8.

49. Mahajan L, Oliva L, Wyllie R, et al. The safety of gastrostomy in patients with Crohn's disease. *Am J Gastroenterol* 1997;92:985–8.

50. Cosgrove M, Jenkins HR. Experience of percutaneous endoscopic gastrostomy in children with Crohn's disease. *Arch Dis Child* 1997;76:141–3.

51. Anstee QM, Forbes A. The safe use of percutaneous gastrostomy for enteral nutrition in patients with Crohn's disease. *Eur J Gastroenterol Hepatol* 2000;12:1089–93.

52. Chun H, Sasaki M, Fujiyama Y, et al. Effect of enteral glutamine on intestinal permeability and bacterial translocation after abdominal radiation injury in rats. *J Gastroenterol* 1997;32:189–95.

53. Soderholm JD, Olaison G, Lindberg E, et al. Different intestinal permeability patterns in relatives and spouses of patients with Crohn's disease: an inherited defect in mucosal defence? *Gut* 1999;44:96–100.

54. Den Hond E, Hiele M, Peeters M, et al. Effect of long-term oral glutamine supplements on small intestinal permeability in patients with Crohn's disease. *JPEN J Parenter Enteral Nutr* 1999;23:7–11.

55. Belluzzi A, Brignola C, Campieri M, et al. Effect of an enteric-coated fish-oil preparation on relapses in Crohn's disease. *N Engl J Med* 1996;334:1557–60.

56. Lorenz R, Weber PC, Szimnau P, et al. Supplementation with n-3 fatty acids from fish oil in chronic inflammatory bowel disease – a randomized, placebo-controlled, double-blind cross-over trial. *J Intern Med Suppl* 1989;225:225–32.

57. Buffinton GD, Doe WF. Depleted mucosal antioxidant defences in inflammatory bowel disease. *Free Radic Biol Med* 1995;19:911–18.

58. Lih-Brody L, Powell SR, Collier KP, et al. Increased oxidative stress and decreased antioxidant defenses in mucosa of inflammatory bowel disease. *Dig Dis Sci* 1996;41:2078–86.

59. Geerling BJ, Badart-Smook A, van Deursen C, et al. Nutritional supplementation with N-3 fatty acids and antioxidants in patients with Crohn's disease in remission: effects on antioxidant status and fatty acid profile. *Inflamm Bowel Dis* 2000;6:77–84.

60. Aghdassi E, Wendland BE, Steinhart AH, et al. Antioxidant vitamin supplementation in Crohn's disease decreases oxidative stress. A randomized controlled trial. *Am J Gastroenterol* 2003;98:348–53.

61. Giaffer MH, Cann P, Holdsworth CD. Long-term effects of elemental and exclusion diets for Crohn's disease. *Aliment Pharmacol Ther* 1991;5:115–25.

62. Pearson M, Teahon K, Levi AJ, et al. Food intolerance and Crohn's disease. *Gut* 1993;34:783–7.

63. Riordan AM, Hunter JO, Cowan RE, et al. Treatment of active Crohn's disease by exclusion diet: East Anglian multicentre controlled trial. *Lancet* 1993;342:1131–4.

64. Lewis JD, Fisher RL. Nutrition support in inflammatory bowel disease. *Med Clin North Am* 1994;78:1443–56.

65. Geerling BJ, Badart-Smook A, Stockbrugger RW, et al. Comprehensive nutritional status in recently diagnosed patients with inflammatory bowel disease compared with population controls. *Eur J Clin Nutr* 2000;54:514–21.

66. McIntyre PB, Powell-Tuck J, Wood SR, et al. Controlled trial of bowel rest in the treatment of severe acute colitis. *Gut* 1986;27:481–5.

67. Dickinson RJ, Ashton MG, Axon AT, et al. Controlled trial of intravenous hyperalimentation and total bowel rest as an adjunct to the routine therapy of acute colitis. *Gastroenterology* 1980;79:1199–1204.

68. Gonzalez-Huix F, Fernandez-Banares F, Esteve-Comas M, et al. Enteral versus parenteral nutrition as adjunct therapy in acute ulcerative colitis. *Am J Gastroenterol* 1993;88:227–32.

69. The Veterans Affairs Total Parenteral Nutrition Cooperative Study Group. Perioperative total parenteral nutrition in surgical patients. *N Engl J Med* 1991;325:525–32.

70. D'Argenio G, Mazzacca G. Short-chain fatty acid in the human colon. Relation to inflammatory bowel diseases and colon cancer. *Adv Exp Med Biol* 1999;472:149–58.

71. Steinhart AH, Hiruki T, Brzezinski A, et al. Treatment of left-sided ulcerative colitis with butyrate enemas: a controlled trial. *Aliment Pharmacol Ther* 1996;10:729–36.

72. Breuer RI, Soergel KH, Lashner BA, et al. Short chain fatty acid rectal irrigation for left-sided ulcerative colitis: a randomised, placebo controlled trial. *Gut* 1997;40:485–91.

73. Scheppach W. Treatment of distal ulcerative colitis with short-chain fatty acid enemas. A placebo-controlled trial. German–Austrian SCFA Study Group. *Dig Dis Sci* 1996;41:2254–9.

74. Hallert C, Bjorck I, Nyman M, et al. Increasing fecal butyrate in ulcerative colitis patients by diet: controlled pilot study. *Inflamm Bowel Dis* 2003;9:116–21.

75. Mitsuyama K, Saiki T, Kanauchi O, et al. Treatment of ulcerative colitis with germinated barley foodstuff feeding: a pilot study. *Aliment Pharmacol Ther* 1998;12:1225–30.

76. Nordgaard I, Hove H, Clausen MR, et al. Colonic production of butyrate in patients with previous colonic cancer during long-term treatment with dietary fibre (*Plantago ovata* seeds). *Scand J Gastroenterol* 1996;31:1011–20.

77. Fernandez-Banares F, Hinojosa J, Sanchez-Lombrana JL, et al. Randomized clinical trial of *Plantago ovata* seeds (dietary fiber) as compared with mesalamine in maintaining remission in ulcerative colitis. Spanish Group for the Study of Crohn's Disease and Ulcerative Colitis (GETECCU). *Am J Gastroenterol* 1999;94:427–33.

78. Stenson WF, Cort D, Rodgers J, et al. Dietary supplementation with fish oil in ulcerative colitis. *Ann Intern Med* 1992;116:609–14.

79. Aslan A, Triadafilopoulos G. Fish oil fatty acid supplementation in active ulcerative colitis: a double-blind, placebo-controlled, crossover study. *Am J Gastroenterol* 1992;87:432–7.

80. Hawthorne AB, Daneshmend TK, Hawkey CJ, et al. Treatment of ulcerative colitis with fish oil supplementation: a prospective 12 month randomised controlled trial. *Gut* 1992;33:922–8.

81. Dichi I, Frenhane P, Dichi JB, et al. Comparison of omega-3 fatty acids and sulfasalazine in ulcerative colitis. *Nutrition* 2000;16:87–90.

82. Lashner BA, Provencher KS, Seidner DL, et al. The effect of folic acid supplementation on the risk for cancer or dysplasia in ulcerative colitis. *Gastroenterology* 1997;112:29–32.

83. Lashner BA, Heidenreich PA, Su GL, et al. Effect of folate supplementation on the incidence of dysplasia and cancer in chronic ulcerative colitis. A case-control study. *Gastroenterology* 1989;97:255–9.

84. Cravo ML, Albuquerque CM, Salazar de Sousa L, et al. Microsatellite instability in non-neoplastic mucosa of patients with ulcerative colitis: effect of folate supplementation. *Am J Gastroenterol* 1998;93:2060–4.

85. Papa A, De Stefano V, Danese S, et al. Hyperhomocysteinemia and prevalence of polymorphisms of homocysteine metabolism-related enzymes in patients with inflammatory bowel disease. *Am J Gastroenterol* 2001;96:2677–82.

86. Nakano E, Taylor CJ, Chada L, et al. Hyperhomocystinemia in children with inflammatory bowel disease. *J Pediatr Gastroenterol Nutr* 2003;37:586–90.

4

Recent advances in surgical management

Robin S McLeod

Introduction

Many inflammatory bowel disease patients require surgery at some point in their disease course. Surgery is potentially curative in patients with ulcerative colitis (UC), while recurrence is common following surgery in patients with Crohn's disease (CD). As a result, the indications for surgery and the surgical decision making may be quite different in the two diseases.

The past 50 years have seen significant advances in the surgical management of UC. Although there are several options available to patients, the preferred option is now the ileal pouch procedure. With technical modifications and experience, this procedure can be performed with a low complication rate, good functional results, and excellent quality of life and long-term outcome.

In CD patients, surgery is usually reserved for the management of complications or for when medical treatment has failed. The usual procedure is resection of the diseased segment. To date, no surgical maneuvers have been shown to decrease the risk of recurrence. Over the past few decades, several advances have been made in the surgical management of CD:

- use of strictureplasty for extensive disease

- use of laparoscopic techniques to perform surgery

- performance of the ileal pouch procedure in highly selected patients

Despite advances in medical therapy, surgery is still required in a large proportion of patients with UC and CD. The need for surgery should not be perceived as a failure of medical therapy. Rather, one should view treatment as multimodal – including both surgical and medical therapies – and each may be required at different points in the disease course.

While the manifestations of and even the surgical procedures performed for UC and CD may be similar, there is a fundamental difference in the surgical approach to these diseases. Because CD is a panintestinal disease, it cannot be eliminated; indeed, recurrence is one of the most important considerations in the management of CD. Thus, surgery is usually limited to managing the complications of the disease. On the other hand, UC can be cured. Therefore, some of the concerns related to surgery for CD do not apply in UC, and improved quality of life is a major goal.

Obviously, surgery for inflammatory bowel disease (IBD) is complex. This chapter concentrates on some of the newer developments and controversial aspects of surgery for IBD.

Surgery for ulcerative colitis

The surgical management of UC has advanced tremendously over the past 50 years, dating back to Bryan Brooke's description of the matured ileostomy, Rupert Turnbull's promotion of the profession of enterostomal therapy, and Nils Kock's pioneering work in continence procedures. In the late 1970s, Parks and Utsunomiya independently adapted the ileal reservoir, which had previously been described by Kock, and anastomosed it to the anus, creating what has become known as a restorative proctocolectomy, ileal pouch-anal anastomosis (IPAA), or pelvic pouch (see **Figure 1**) [1,2]. Its major advantage over other procedures is that the normal

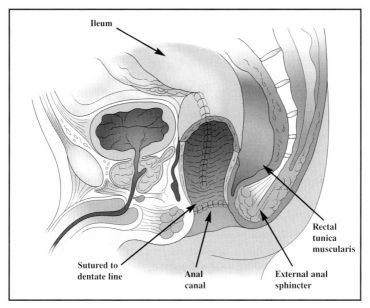

Figure 1. Diagram of ileoanal pouch anastomosis. Reproduced from Ehrenpreis, ED. *Anal and Rectal Diseases Explained*. London: Remedica Publishing, 2003.

route of evacuation is maintained and the need for a permanent ileostomy is eliminated. This has become the procedure of choice for most patients requiring surgery for UC.

Patient selection

Older age

Older age is a relative contraindication. However, even this is being challenged as the complication rate for surgery decreases. Delaney, from the Cleveland Clinic, reported on IPAA in 42 patients >65 years old. When compared with a group of younger patients, the complication rate in the older patients was not significantly increased, although incontinence and night-time seepage were more common in the older age group and quality of life was somewhat lower [3]. However, 89% of individuals in the >65-years group were happy that they had had surgery, and 96% would recommend it to others.

When IPAA is performed in elderly patients, it is important to individualize decisions, especially if the patient has significant comorbidities. If a patient is not a candidate for IPAA, then data suggest that quality of life is excellent in most patients with a total proctocolectomy, although functional results may be less predictable in this age group.

Perianal disease

Perianal disease is a relative contraindication to performing a reconstructive procedure because of concern that the patient may have CD; also, there may be a higher risk of anastomotic complications. Richard et al. reported on 49 patients who had perianal disease and underwent a IPAA procedure [4]. Although the anastomotic complication rate was higher in this cohort of patients, the pouch failure rate was not increased. This suggests that in selected patients where the suspicion of CD is low, and where the perianal disease has been treated, an IPAA procedure can be considered.

Cancer

If UC is complicated by cancer, a pouch operation can usually be performed if the cancer is located in the colon and the patient desires the operation. However, if the patient has advanced cancer and his lifespan may be shortened, it might be prudent to do a more limited procedure as short-term outcomes may be bad. In addition, patients with low-lying rectal cancer may require a total proctocolectomy. Surgical cancer principles should not be compromised in order to perform a reconstructive procedure. A pouch procedure may also not be feasible if the patient requires postoperative radiation.

Although the risk of developing a postoperative cancer in the rectal cuff is extremely remote, almost all of the reported cancers have occurred in patients who had a cancer or dysplasia at the time of the colectomy. Thus, if a pouch procedure is performed, patients should be made aware of this small, but nevertheless increased, risk of cancer.

Staged procedures

Finally, there is a role for staged procedures in some patients. Patients whose nutritional status is suboptimal, who have acute or fulminant colitis and are on high doses of steroids, or whose diagnosis is in doubt should initially have a subtotal colectomy, subsequently followed by a proctectomy and pouch procedure. Since many surgeons are now performing the pouch procedure in patients who have had a previous colectomy, without a defunctioning ileostomy, this may be a sensible option and does not mean that the patient will require a three-stage procedure.

Technical considerations

The IPAA procedure is technically difficult. When it was first introduced, complication rates of 60%–70% and failure rates of up to 30% were reported. The complication rate has since decreased dramatically, and the overall failure rate is now <5% in reported series [5–7]. This is due to modifications in technique as well as increased experience with both the technical aspects of the procedure and the management of complications.

Several types of pouches have been described, including the S, J, and W pouches. Of these, the J pouch is most commonly performed because of its ease of construction (see **Figure 2**). There does not appear to be any long-term advantage of one design over the others. In the short-term, the pouch capacity may be larger with the W- or S-shaped pouches [8].

The most significant change in technique has been dissection of the rectum to the level of the levators followed by construction of a stapled ileoanal anastomosis (IAA) approximately 1–2 cm above the dentate line, rather than performing a mucosectomy and hand-sewn anastomosis. Again, the major advantage is a technical one. In obese individuals and in heavy-set males, it may be extremely difficult to bring the pouch down to the anal outlet to do a hand-sewn anastomosis. There are also some data to suggest that functional results may be improved and that the anastomotic leak rate is lower with a stapled anastomosis [5,9,10]. A concern with

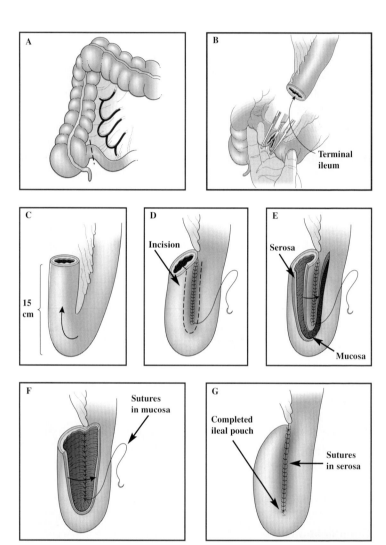

Figure 2. Construction of a J-shaped ileal pouch. (**A,B**) The terminal ileum is divided and the colon is removed. (**C**) The terminal ileum is fashioned into a J-shape with 15-cm limbs. (**D,E**) The antimesenteric border of the ileum is divided. (**F**) The posterior mucosal layer of the pouch is sutured. (**G**) The pouch is completed. Reproduced from Ehrenpreis, ED. *Anal and Rectal Diseases Explained*. London: Remedica Publishing, 2003.

leaving the short cuff of rectal mucosa is that there may be continued symptoms due to inflammation, or the development of cancer. Although inflammation persists in this segment of mucosa, symptomatic "cuffitis" requiring medical or surgical therapy is rare. With regards to the development of cancer in the anal outlet, there have been some reported cases, but these have occurred with similar frequency in individuals who have had a mucosectomy as in those who have had a stapled anastomosis.

In the initial descriptions of the procedure, a defunctioning stoma was always performed. However, as leak rates have decreased, some surgeons now routinely omit the ileostomy while others do so on a selective basis [5,11]. At our institution, an ileostomy is omitted if the patient has previously had a subtotal colectomy and is therefore off all steroids and nutritionally fit, and if a double-stapled IAA is performed.

The other, more recent change in technique has been to perform pouch surgery laparoscopically. Centers performing laparoscopic pouches do so in very selected patients. Marcello and Milsom published a series of 20 patients who had the procedure performed laparoscopically. A Pfannenstiel incision was made to transect the rectum and construct the pouch. These patients were matched to 20 patients who were operated on with an open technique – operative time was longer in the laparoscopic cases (330 minutes for laparoscopic cases vs 230 minutes for open cases), but length of stay (7 vs 8 days) and complication rates (20% vs 25%) were similar [12].

Complications

Postoperative deaths are extremely rare, and a low complication rate can be achieved in experienced hands. Heuschen et al. analyzed various risk factors in their series of >700 patients who had undergone an ileal pouch procedure [13]. They found that UC patients who were receiving >40 mg/day of prednisone had a significantly higher risk of septic complications. Anastomotic tension was a factor in patients with familial adenomatous polyposis.

The most serious early complication is a leak from the IAA. This may manifest as a radiological leak, a clinical leak with an intra-abdominal abscess, a fistula to another intra-abdominal structure, a perianal abscess, or a fistula to the perineum or vagina. A leak most frequently manifests within a few days of the procedure, but may occur many months after the procedure or closure of the ileostomy. The reported risk of an anastomotic leak is quite variable, ranging from 5% to 15%. Experience of the surgeon is a factor, and the IAA leak rate has decreased over time.

Staging of the procedure may affect the leak rate. In a small early series, high leak rates were reported in patients who had the procedure performed without a covering ileostomy [14]. At our center, we omit ileostomy in patients who have previously had a subtotal colectomy and ileostomy [5]. This is based on an initial experience of 71 patients who had an IPAA procedure without a defunctioning ileostomy and in whom the leak rate was 18%. Those who had the procedure as a single stage had a leak rate of 32% compared with only 12% in those who had a previous subtotal colectomy. Similarly, those on steroids had a higher leak rate (33% vs 14%). Other centers, however, continue to perform IPAA without a covering ileostomy and report adequate results [11].

It also seems that a hand-sewn anastomosis is associated with a higher rate of leaks than a stapled anastomosis. Ziv et al. reported a septic complication rate of 10.5% in those having a hand-sewn IPAA compared with 4.6% in those having a stapled IPAA [10].

Anastomotic leaks are significant not only because of their frequency, but also because they are the most common reason for pouch excision. In those in whom the pouch is not excised, functional results may be impaired. In our series of 58 patients requiring excision of the pouch, 39% of excisions were because of a leak from the IAA and 12% because of a leak from the pouch itself [15]. Gemlo reported that perianal sepsis or pouch fistulas were the cause of failure in 24% of their patients who required excision of the pouch [16].

In the 1980s, a leak most often led to excision of the pouch, but as experience with the procedure and with the management of complications has increased, most pouches can be salvaged. Various modalities can be used, including antibiotics and drainage of the pouch (if there is no covering ileostomy), delayed closure of the ileostomy, local techniques for repair of the anastomosis, and reconstruction of the pouch with a combined abdominoperineal approach. By utilizing these various management options, 75%–85% of pouches can be salvaged [17–19].

Although construction of an ileostomy may be important to decrease the morbidity from an anastomotic leak, the ileostomy itself may be a source of morbidity [20]. The most common complication is dehydration secondary to high ileostomy outputs. Usually, dietary maneuvers, antidiarrheal agents, and fluid replacement will be sufficient treatment. Rarely, early closure of the ileostomy is required. However, this is not a major complication and does not impact on the long-term outcome. Surgical complications occurring after closure of the ileostomy, such as an anastomotic leak, fistula, or obstruction, are much more significant and occur in up to 5% of patients.

Small bowel obstruction continues to be a major source of morbidity. In our own series, approximately 30% of patients required at least one admission for the management of small bowel obstruction by 10 years, although <10% required reoperation [21].

The risk of pouch failure has also decreased over time. The currently reported failure rates are approximately 5%. MacRae reported on an early series of 551 patients in whom the failure rate was 10.5% [15]. The risk factors for failure were hand-sewn IAA, tension on the IAA, use of a defunctioning ileostomy, CD, and a leak from the pouch or IAA. Gemlo reported a failure rate of 9.9% in 253 patients having surgery at the University of Minnesota [16]. A poor functional result was the most common cause (28%), followed by unsuspected CD (5%) and pelvic sepsis. Lepisto reported an overall failure rate of 5.3% [7]. The cumulative probability of pouch failure was 1% at 1 year, 5% at 5 years, and 7% at 10 years. Fistula was a predictor of failure.

Long-term complications and outcome
Pouchitis
Pouchitis is a complication unique to pouches [22]. It is a nonspecific inflammation that manifests as increased stool frequency, pain in the lower abdomen, and, occasionally, low-grade fever. On endoscopy, the pouch is acutely inflamed with evidence of friability, ulceration, and mucous discharge. On histology, there should be evidence of acute inflammation to make the diagnosis of pouchitis. The cumulative risk of pouchitis may be as high as 30%–50% at 5 years [23]. Fortunately, most episodes begin abruptly and respond quickly to antibiotics, even though the etiology of pouchitis is unknown. Pouchitis is chronic in only a few percent of individuals, with patients requiring long-term antibiotic therapy, and only 1% will require pouch excision.

Antibiotics are the mainstay of treatment [24]. Other treatments – such as bismuth, allopurinol, glutamine, and cyclosporine enemas – have been tried, but are of little benefit. There are some data to suggest that probiotics may be beneficial in preventing pouchitis and maintaining remission in those who have had pouchitis [25,26].

Cancer and dysplasia
There has been concern as to whether there is an increased risk of cancer and dysplasia in individuals who have had an IPAA procedure. Potentially, both the residual rectal mucosa and the pouch mucosa are at risk. Several cases of cancer have been reported in the rectal mucosa. These have occurred in individuals in whom a mucosectomy was performed, as well as in

those where a mucosectomy was omitted [27–35]. Most, however, have occurred in individuals who had a cancer or dysplasia in the colectomy specimen. Regular endoscopy and biopsy of the remaining rectal mucosa should be performed in individuals with a history of UC of >10 years duration.

While there have been a few reported cases of cancer and dysplasia affecting the pouch mucosa, it is still uncertain whether the risk of cancer is increased in this cohort of patients [36–42]. If there is an increased risk, it may be in patients with chronic pouchitis with severe villous atrophy on histology [36].

Sexual dysfunction and infertility
Males undergoing pelvic surgery are at risk for injury to the pelvic nerves. This may result in difficulty emptying the bladder, retrograde ejaculation, or impotence. These symptoms may occur transiently or permanently, and may be partial or complete. When surgery is being performed for UC, it is unnecessary to perform a wide pelvic dissection; therefore, the risk should be significantly lower than in patients having surgery for rectal cancer. Nevertheless, the reported risk is approximately 1%–2%.

Recently, studies have documented an increased risk of infertility in females having a pelvic procedure. The ability to conceive may be decreased by 50% [43]. The mechanism by which this occurs is unknown, but is probably related to adhesion formation following pelvic surgery. On the other hand, women who do become pregnant do not seem to have problems with either the pregnancy or delivery. The risk of perineal complications is not increased nor are functional results permanently impaired, so the decision whether to have a vaginal delivery or cesarean section may be left to the woman and her obstetrician [44,45].

Quality of life
Quality of life is an important issue in assessing the outcome of surgery for UC, since in most patients the indication for surgery

is failure of medical management or poor quality of life. Although the IPAA procedure is preferred by most patients, there are data to suggest that quality of life is excellent irrespective of the surgical procedure performed, possibly because physical well-being, which is the main determinant of outcome, is improved [46]. Various validated instruments, including utility assessments and psychometric instruments such as the short form-36 and inflammatory bowel disease questionnaire, have been used to measure quality of life pre- and postoperatively [47,48]. Multiple studies have shown that quality of life is improved postoperatively and is similar to that observed in the "normal" population.

Surgery for Crohn's disease

General issues

In many patients with CD, surgery is indicated to treat a septic complication. Indeed, abdominal abscesses may complicate CD in 10%–28% of patients. With advances in imaging, especially computed tomography scans, and the ability to manage abscesses nonoperatively, the management of patients with septic complications has changed considerably [49,50]. Most patients will ultimately require surgery, but percutaneous drainage of the abscess decreases the morbidity of the operation and obviates the need for a temporary stoma.

Gervais et al. reported their experience in 32 patients with CD, in whom 53 abscesses were drained [50]. This included 19 patients who had spontaneous abscesses and 13 in whom an abscess occurred postoperatively. The abscesses were drained successfully 96% of the time. In the 19 patients who had abscesses related to their disease process, 69% avoided surgery within the first month following abscess drainage. The presence of a fistula was a predictor of success: 80% of patients with a documented fistula required early surgery compared with 36% of patients in whom a fistula was not visualized. However, in the long-term, only 15% of patients with a spontaneous abscess did not require surgical intervention for their CD.

Corticosteroid dosing

A major indication for surgery is failure of medical therapy. As a result, most patients will be on some form of medication preoperatively and these drugs could potentially impact on surgery. There may be concerns related to healing in patients who are on high doses of steroids. Depending on the dose of steroids and the general status of the patient, it may be prudent to delay performing an anastomosis or a temporary defunctioning stoma proximal to the anastomosis.

Brown and Buie reviewed the literature regarding the need for perioperative steroid coverage in patients who were either taking or had a history of taking steroids [51]. They concluded that there is no evidence that supraphysiologic doses of corticosteroids are necessary to prevent hemodynamic instability secondary to adrenal insufficiency in the perioperative period. They recommended that patients who are on steroids preoperatively should continue on the same dose of steroids throughout the perioperative period. Only critically ill patients requiring vasopressors should be started on high doses of steroids and at the same time be tested for adrenal insufficiency.

Infliximab

Brezezinski et al. reviewed the Cleveland Clinic surgical experience with 35 patients who received infliximab in the perioperative period [52]. A total of 22 patients received infliximab preoperatively and 13 postoperatively. Surgery and complications were classified as major or minor. Although this was a small series, there did not appear to be an increased risk of surgical complications in these patients compared with a group of historical controls.

Azathioprine

There are few data to suggest that azathioprine has a deleterious effect on surgical outcome and hence it generally does not need to be stopped preoperatively.

Laparoscopic surgery

The introduction of laparoscopic techniques has had a major impact on surgery for CD. Patients have been enthusiastic about this approach because of the improved cosmetic result and decreased postoperative pain. On the other hand, there is no consistent evidence that hospital stays are shortened significantly or that return to work occurs earlier following laparoscopy. As laparoscopic techniques have become more widely adopted, the indications have widened. Laparoscopic resections may be more difficult in patients who have had previous surgery and in those who have multiple adhesions or a large inflammatory mass, abscess, or fistula. Nevertheless, most procedures in CD patients can now be attempted laparoscopically and converted to an open procedure if necessary.

The laparoscopic approach for performing defunctioning stomas offers real advantages over an open approach. It is easy to perform, with the stoma being brought out through one of the port sites. Currently, terminal ileal and right colon resections, segmental resections of the small and large bowel, proctectomy, and reconstruction of the gastrointestinal tract following a Hartmann procedure are all being performed laparoscopically. Most proponents advocate performing laparoscopic-assisted resections so that the bowel is exteriorized through a small incision at one of the port sites, and the mesentery, which is often thickened, is divided extracorporally.

Some studies have compared the results of laparoscopic ileocolic resection with either historical or concurrent controls who had open surgery [53–56]. In these studies, the complication rates were generally comparable, at approximately 10%. However, the length of hospital stay was significantly decreased, with savings of 2–5 days in the laparoscopic group. As a result of this, two studies reported savings in direct hospital costs [57,58].

Only one randomized controlled trial has compared open with laparoscopic ileocolic resection. Milsom et al. randomized

31 patients to a laparoscopic group and 29 to conventional surgery [59]. The times to flatus and first bowel movement did not differ significantly. The median length of stay was 5 days after laparoscopic and 6 days after conventional surgery. There was no significant difference in the rate of major complications, but there were significantly more minor complications in the conventional surgery group. Two patients in the laparoscopic group were converted to an open procedure because of adhesions or inflammation.

Surgery for small bowel and ileocolic CD

Although CD may affect any part of the small bowel, the terminal ileum is most frequently involved. At the other end of the spectrum, there may be multiple skip lesions throughout the small bowel. The pattern of disease may also vary, with patients having primarily fibrostenotic, inflammatory, or fistulizing disease. Depending on the site of the disease and indication for surgery, the surgical approach may vary. However, resection remains the preferred option in most patients with small bowel or ileocolic disease. Although strictureplasty is used in only selected patients, it has been a valuable addition to the surgical armamentarium in CD.

Bypass procedures (the "Eisenhower procedure") were popular in the 1960s, but they are now rarely performed because of the high rate of recrudescence of the disease in the short-term and the increased risk of small bowel cancer in the long-term. At present, the only indication for a bypass procedure would be a gastrojejunostomy for duodenal CD. In the unusual situation where the surgeon feels it is unsafe to resect small intestinal disease, a defunctioning ileostomy would be preferable to a bypass procedure. However, this situation is now rarely encountered because of improved imaging techniques and the ability to percutaneously drain abscesses preoperatively.

Bowel resection
Surgical resection results in improved well-being and quality of life in most patients. However, recurrence of disease following

surgery remains a major concern. Recurrence rates vary depending on whether the criteria used to define recurrence are endoscopic, clinical, or need for further surgery [60]. Endoscopic recurrence rates varying from 29% to 93% at 1 year have been reported [60–63]. The clinical or symptomatic recurrence rates, which are probably most relevant, have been reported to range from 6% to 16% per year [60]. In a population-based cohort of 907 subjects who had ileocecal resections, Bernell et al. reported clinical relapse rates of 28% at 5 years and 36% at 10 years following resection [64].

Various surgical maneuvers have been proposed to decrease the risk of recurrence. The data pertaining to the effect of microscopic disease at the resection margin come from retrospective case studies. The data are conflicting [65]. However, given that CD is a panintestinal disease, that it is focal in distribution, and that histological abnormalities have been demonstrated in segments of bowel that appear to be grossly normal, the significance of microscopic disease at the resection margin is questionable.

The length of the resection margin has also generated differing and controversial results. However, there is level I evidence that longer resection margins do not result in a lower risk of recurrence. Fazio et al. randomized 152 patients to a group with proximal resection margins of 2 cm in length or another with proximal resection margins of 12 cm in length [66]. After a mean follow-up of 56 months, the recurrence rate (as defined by the need for a further resection) was 25% in the limited resection group compared with 18% in the extended resection group (not statistically significant). Thus, the approach accepted by most surgeons is to resect the bowel that is grossly involved, plus a margin of several centimeters of normal bowel.

There are conflicting data on whether the type of anastomosis alters the risk of recurrence. Two trials have addressed this issue. Cameron et al. randomized 86 patients who had an ileocolic resection to an end-to-end anastomosis or end-to-side anastomosis [67]. After a mean follow-up of 47 months, the recurrence rates in the two groups were similar at 23% and 31%, respectively. Ikeuchi et al. randomized 33 patients to a hand-sewn end-to-end anastomosis and 30 patients to a stapled functional end-to-end (using the 60-mm linear stapler) or circular-stapled anastomosis [68]. There were a variety of anastomotic sites, including ileoileal, ileocolic, colocolic, and ileorectal anastomoses. Recurrence was defined as the need for another operation because of disease recurrence. The recurrence rate was significantly lower in the stapled group compared with the hand-sewn group (18.9% vs 37.8%) after a median follow-up of 87 months.

It is hypothesized that a side-to-side anastomosis may be wider and therefore leads to less fecal stasis than an end-to-end anastomosis. There are no randomized controlled trials comparing side-to-side and end-to-end anastomoses. Munoz-Juarez et al. reviewed the experience of 138 patients who had ileocolic resections at the Mayo Clinic and Birmingham General Hospital [69]. Sixty-nine patients who had stapled side-to-side anastomoses were age and gender matched to 69 patients who had end-to-end sutured anastomoses. The groups were similar with the exception of mean follow-up (20 vs 35 months), which may account for the difference in the symptomatic recurrence rates of 18% in the stapled group and 48% in the sutured group. Two further studies have reported similar findings [70,71]. On the other hand, two other studies found no difference in recurrence rates when the data were analyzed actuarially [72,73]. The discrepancies in these reports may be because they were retrospective, with variable criteria for diagnosing recurrence and anastomotic techniques and differing follow-ups.

Strictureplasty

Strictureplasty was first advocated in the 1980s for the treatment of fibrotic strictures in CD [74]. Two types of strictureplasty have been described: the Heineke Mikulicz, which is performed for short strictures, and the Finney, which is performed for longer strictures. Michelassi et al. described a side-to-side isoperistaltic strictureplasty for the management of a long segment of disease or multiple strictures in the mid small bowel [75]. In this procedure, the bowel is divided and a side-to-side anastomosis is performed, thus avoiding a resection, blind loop, or bypassed segment. Their report documents the results in 21 patients. One patient had a postoperative bleed. After follow-up of up to 7.5 years, there was evidence of disease regression in all patients. Another report from Poggioli et al. described a strictureplasty where a side-to-side anastomosis was performed between the diseased terminal ileum and the right colon [76]. This technique has been used in only five patients and therefore its utility has yet to be determined.

Despite the concerns of anastomosing diseased bowel, the short-term complication rates following strictureplasty are low, with reported complication rates ranging from 1% to 14% [77]. The Cleveland Clinic reported their experience with 1,224 strictureplasties in 314 patients [78]. With a median follow-up of 7.5 years, 34% of their patients have required further surgery for symptomatic CD. Hurst and Michelassi reported a recurrence of disease necessitating reoperation of 15 ± 6% at 1 year and 22 ± 10% at 5 years [79].

Given that the procedure can be performed safely and that a conservative approach to CD is advocated, strictureplasty has an important role in the surgical management of patients with CD. However, at the present time, its use is generally limited to those patients who have multiple skip lesions or who have had multiple resections previously. Tichansky reported that obstruction was the indication for surgery in 92% of patients [77]. It is contraindicated in patients with long strictures, abscesses, or fistulizing disease. Although some proponents have suggested that strictureplasty should replace resection in patients with limited disease, the Oxford group reported on a cohort of patients who had surgery for CD; strictureplasty significantly predicted the need for further surgery [80].

Another question that remains unanswered is whether these patients should receive maintenance therapy. There are no data from randomized controlled trials, and opinion seems to be divided on this question. However, since most of these patients have extensive disease, it has recently been our practice to advise prophylaxis with an immunosuppressive such as azathioprine.

Surgery for large bowel disease

The pattern of involvement in Crohn's colitis is quite variable, with some patients having predominantly right-sided involvement (possibly with small bowel involvement), others having colonic involvement with sparing of the rectum, and others having pancolitis. Furthermore, the disease may be complicated by the presence of perianal disease. As a result, both the indications for surgery and the surgical procedure itself may vary. Most patients who require surgery for colonic disease will need a resection. If there is sparing of the rectum and no or minimal perianal disease then a colectomy and ileorectal or ileosigmoid anastomosis can be performed. Proctocolectomy and ileostomy will be required for patients with pancolitis or those with severe perianal disease. The obvious advantage of performing an anastomosis is that a stoma is avoided. However, the reported recurrence rates are significantly higher in patients in whom a colectomy and an anastomosis are performed. Andrews et al. reported recurrence rates of 46% and 60% at 5 and 10 years, respectively, in patients who had ileorectal anastomoses, compared with rates of 10% and 21% in those who had a proctocolectomy and ileostomy [81]. Patients with limited disease of the colon may have a segmental resection. Strictureplasty is rarely an option for patients with Crohn's colitis.

Farmer et al. reported that the indications for surgery in patients with colonic CD were poor response to medical therapy in 26%, presence of an internal fistula and abscesses in 23%, toxic megacolon in 20%, and perianal disease in 19% [82]. Andersson et al. reported on changes in the surgical management of CD in Sweden between 1970 and 1997. There were 211 patients followed during this time, of whom 84 underwent surgery. Indications for and outcome of surgery were compared during the time periods 1977–1990 and 1991–1997 [83]. In the earlier time period, active disease was the indication for surgery in 64% of patients compared with only 25% in the more recent time period. Alongside this, there was a concomitant increase in stricture as the indication for surgery (9% vs 50%). In addition, the median time from diagnosis to operation increased significantly from 3.5 to 11.5 years between the two time periods. The use of proctocolectomy or colectomy as the primary procedure fell from 69% to 10%, whereas segmental resection increased from 31% to 90%. Only 7% of patients were on postoperative maintenance therapy in the early time period compared with 70% more recently.

Colectomy and ileorectal anastomosis
Despite the higher recurrence rates, colectomy and ileorectal anastomosis (IRA) have an important role in the management of CD patients, since many patients are young and would prefer to avoid ileostomy. However, patients must be carefully selected. Those with significant perianal disease or severe rectal disease are not candidates. Longo et al. reviewed 131 patients who underwent colectomy and IRA at the Cleveland Clinic. They found that the presence of small bowel disease preoperatively was the only predictive factor for the need for further surgery [84]. Age at surgery, duration of disease, steroid use, presence of proctitis, and perianal disease did not affect outcome. However, it is quite likely that this was a highly selected group of patients and that those with significant rectal or perianal disease would not have been included. From the results of reported series, it can be anticipated that disease will recur in approximately 50%–65% of patients. In some patients, the recurrence may be confined to the small bowel, making a further resection and anastomosis possible. Thus, approximately 75% of patients may have a functioning IRA at 5 years, and 50% of patients at 10 years.

Proctocolectomy

Proctocolectomy is the procedure of choice for patients with pancolitis or extensive perianal disease. In those with perianal disease with associated sepsis, it may be prudent to perform a subtotal colectomy and ileostomy, and subsequently perform the proctectomy when the sepsis has settled. This may minimize the risk of an unhealed perineal wound. This is the major complication of this operation, and has been reported to occur in up to 20% of patients. Pelvic nerve injury is a rare, but important, complication. As stated previously, the recurrence rates following proctocolectomy and ileostomy are lower than with colectomy and IRA.

Pelvic pouches

Most patients undergoing an IPAA procedure have UC, with a smaller number having familial adenomatous polyposis. However, since the procedure can now be performed with low morbidity and mortality and very good long-term outcome, the indications have widened. The role of IPAA in patients with CD remains controversial. CD has been considered a contraindication because of the risk of small bowel and perianal involvement. Only one report has suggested that the procedure can be performed safely in patients with CD with a failure rate of 7%, similar to that in patients with UC [85]. Although this report suggests that selected CD patients may have a satisfactory outcome with a pouch procedure, one must be somewhat cautious in the interpretation of these results. Since perianal disease frequently complicates CD, these patients are a highly selected group or, alternatively, may have indeterminate colitis. Furthermore, higher failure rates, ranging from 30% to 50%, have been reported by others [86–88]. Thus, CD generally remains a contraindication to performing a pouch procedure. However, this procedure may be considered in patients where disease is limited to the colon and rectum.

Patients must be carefully selected and fully informed that their risk of complications and failure may be higher. Although the complication rate appears to be higher in patients with indeterminate colitis, most surgeons do not consider this a contraindication to performing a pouch procedure [89–91]. Yu et al. from the Mayo Clinic found the pouch failure rate to be significantly higher in patients with indeterminate colitis compared with UC (27% vs 11%) [89]. However, the higher failure rate was observed in patients whose diagnosis was subsequently changed to CD. Thus, it seems that care should be taken to exclude patients with CD to optimize results. A staged procedure with initial subtotal colectomy to allow pathologic examination may be preferred if the diagnosis of UC is in doubt.

Perianal disease

There is a wide range of perianal manifestations, including skin lesions, anal canal lesions, abscesses, and fistulas (see **Figure 3**) [92]. Of these, abscesses and fistulas are of greatest significance to the patient and the most challenging to manage. Often, both medical and surgical modalities must be employed. Initial treatment will depend on the symptoms, the complexity of the fistula, and whether there is associated rectal disease.

Abscesses always require drainage. They should be suspected in patients who have perianal disease and who complain of pain in previously asymptomatic fissures and fistulas. In these patients, one should not hesitate to perform an examination under anesthesia. This may be helpful in assessing the extent of disease and determining whether there is an abscess. Treatment should consist of incision, unroofing, and drainage of abscesses. Primary fistulotomy should usually be avoided. There is no role for treating abscesses with antibiotics alone, although combination metronidazole and ciprofloxacin therapy may be a useful adjunct to surgical drainage, especially if cellulitis is present. Transanal ultrasonography and magnetic resonance imaging may be helpful in patients where the abscess is not obvious, or in delineating the abnormalities in patients with complex disease [93–97].

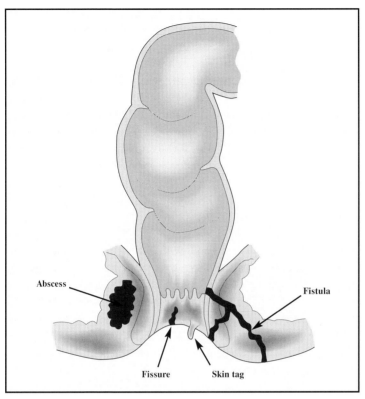

Figure 3. Anorectal disorders seen in patients with Crohn's disease. Reproduced from Ehrenpreis, ED. *Anal and Rectal Diseases Explained*. London: Remedica Publishing, 2003.

Fistulotomy

Simple fistulas are generally amenable to fistulotomy. The fistula can usually be eradicated without risk of incontinence or delayed wound healing. Complex fistulas (including fistulas with multiple external openings or tracts, as well as those that are high) or fistulas occurring in the presence of active rectal disease must be approached differently. Complete surgical eradication is unusual and, where it does occur, significant morbidity generally occurs (especially problems with continence). Before undertaking any form of therapy, an examination should be performed with the patient anesthetized to carefully evaluate the extent of disease and the presence of associated sepsis. Previously undetected abscesses may be drained and tracts can be identified, unroofed, and curetted of all infected granulation tissue. Drains and setons can be inserted on a long-term basis to allow drainage and prevent reaccumulation of pus. Even if healing does not occur, prolonged palliation may be obtained; if necessary, local surgical measures may be repeated. Once the sepsis has been eradicated, one approach is to transpose the internal opening of the fistula tract distally to simplify definitive surgical therapy or perform a flap advancement procedure. Although the results of these techniques are encouraging, the number of patients in each series has been small [98–100].

Medical therapy

Where definitive surgical therapy is not possible or advisable, medical therapy may be an alternative. Most medical therapies, such as antibiotics and immunosuppressives, are of little benefit in healing perianal disease. The major role of antibiotics is to control sepsis and thus minimize the symptoms. Anti-tumor necrosis factor may prove to be an effective medical therapy, particularly for perianal fistulas. Present et al. performed a Phase III randomized controlled trial of 94 adult patients with abdominal or perianal fistulas who were randomized to infliximab 5 mg/kg, infliximab 10 mg/kg, or placebo [101]. Almost 90% of the patients included in the trial had perianal fistulas. There was complete healing of 38%–55% of fistulas in the infliximab groups compared with 13% of patients in the placebo group.

Van Bodegraven et al. reported a series of eight patients with perianal and vaginal or perineal fistulas treated with infliximab. Despite clinical evidence of improvement, all of the patients had ultrasonographic evidence of the fistulous tracts [102]. Poritz et al. reported complete or partial improvement with infliximab in 18 of 26 patients with fistulas (69%), although more than half of them went on to require surgery with a mean follow-up of 6 months [103]. Infliximab appeared to be most effective in treating perianal fistulas, with only four out of nine patients (44%) requiring surgery. Obviously, longer-term follow-up will be required to fully determine the role of infliximab. Infliximab may decrease the drainage from fistulas, as do antibiotics, but fail to cause complete healing of the fistulas. If so, long-term outcomes may not be changed. Should medical measures fail, be refused by a patient, or be contraindicated, patients may require more definitive surgery with a loop ileostomy or proctectomy.

Rectovaginal fistulas

The presence of a rectovaginal fistula is often an ominous sign indicating severe rectal disease. Thus, in most instances, proctectomy or proximal diversion is necessary. However, in very selected patients, local repair of the fistula may be undertaken. Medical treatment alone is usually unsuccessful in the treatment of these fistulas because it is a short tract that epithelializes. Spontaneous closure is also very rare. Medical treatment may have a role in inducing a remission of the rectal disease so that a local repair can be undertaken, or in improving the consistency of stool so that there is less discharge through the fistula opening.

Treatment depends on two factors: patient symptoms and the disease status of the rectum. If the fistula is small and low lying, the patient may experience relatively minor symptoms and no treatment is indicated (other than medical management of any rectal disease). However, if the patient has persistent fecal or purulent discharge from the vagina or gross incontinence, treatment is indicated. Local repair of the fistula should be undertaken only when the disease is in remission and the rectal tissue is healthy. Healing may be expected in 50%–60% of patients [104].

References

1. Parks AG, Nicholls RJ, Belliveau P. Proctocolectomy with ileal reservoir and anal anastomosis. *Br J Surg* 1980;67:533–8.
2. Utsunomiya J, Iwama T, Imajo M, et al. Total colectomy, mucosal proctectomy, and ileoanal anastomosis. *Dis Colon Rectum* 1980;23:459–66.
3. Delaney CP, Fazio VW, Remzi FH, et al. Prospective, age-related analysis of surgical results, functional outcome, and quality of life after ileal pouch-anal anastomosis. *Ann Surg* 2003;238:221–8.
4. Richard CS, Cohen Z, Stern HS, et al. Outcome of the IPAA procedure in patients with prior perianal disease. *Dis Colon Rectum* 1997;40:647–52.
5. Cohen Z, McLeod RS, Stephen W, et al. Continuing evolution of the IPAA procedure. *Ann Surg* 1992;216:506–11; discussion 511–12.
6. Fazio VW, Ziv Y, Church JM, et al. Ileal pouch-anal anastomosis complications and function in 1005 patients. *Ann Surg* 1995;222:120–7.
7. Lepisto A, Luukkonen P, Jarvinen HJ. Cumulative failure rate of ileal pouch-anal anastomosis and quality of life after failure. *Dis Colon Rectum* 2002;45:1289–94.
8. Nicholls RJ, Pezim ME. Restorative proctocolectomy with ileal reservoir for ulcerative colitis and familial adenomatous polyposis: a comparison of three reservoir designs. *Br J Surg* 1985;72:470–4.
9. Johnston D, Holdsworth PJ, Nasmyth DG, et al. Preservation of the entire anal canal in conservation proctocolectomy for ulcerative colitis: a pilot study without mucosal resection with mucosal proctectomy and endo-anal anastomosis. *Br J Surg* 1987;74:940–4.
10. Ziv Y, Fazio VW, Church JM, et al. Stapled ileal pouch anal anastomoses are safer than handsewn anastomoses in patients with ulcerative colitis. *Am J Surg* 1996;171:320–3.
11. Sugerman HJ, Newsome HH. Stapled ileoanal anastomosis without a temporary ileostomy. *Am J Surg* 1994;167:58–65; discussion 65–6.
12. Marcello PW, Milsom JW, Wong SK, et al. Laparoscopic restorative proctocolectomy: case-matched comparative study with open restorative proctocolectomy. *Dis Colon Rectum* 2000;43:604–8.
13. Heuschen UA, Hinz U, Allemeyer EH, et al. Risk factors for ileoanal J pouch-related septic complications in ulcerative colitis and familial adenomatous polyposis. *Ann Surg* 2002;235:207–16.
14. Rothenberger DA, Vermeulen FD, Christenson CE, et al. Restorative proctocolectomy with ileal reservoir and ileoanal anastomosis. *Am J Surg* 1983;145:82–8.
15. MacRae HM, McLeod RS, Cohen Z, et al. Risk factors for IPAA failure. *Dis Colon Rectum* 1997;40:257–62.
16. Gemlo BT, Wong WD, Rothenberger DA, et al. Ileal pouch-anal anastomosis. Patterns of failure. *Arch Surg* 1992;127:784–6; discussion 787.
17. MacLean AR, O'Connor B, Parkes R, et al. Reconstructive surgery for failed ileal pouch-anal anastomosis: a viable surgical option with acceptable results. *Dis Colon Rectum* 2002;45:880–6.
18. Fazio VW, Wu JS, Lavery IC. Repeat ileal pouch-anal anastomosis to salvage septic complications of pelvic pouches: clinical outcome and quality of life assessment. *Ann Surg* 1998;228:588–97.
19. Herbst F, Sielezneff I, Nicholls RJ. Salvage surgery for ileal pouch outlet obstruction *Br J Surg* 1996;83:368–71.
20. Feinberg SM, McLeod RS, Cohen Z. Complications of loop ileostomy. *Am J Surg* 1987;153:102–7.

21. MacLean AR, Cohen Z, MacRae HM, et al. Risk of small bowel obstruction following ileal pouch anastomosis. *Ann Surg* 2002;235:200–6.

22. Sandborn WJ, Tremaine WJ, Batts KP, et al. Pouchitis following ileal pouch-anal anastomosis: a Pouchitis Disease Activity Index. *Mayo Clin Proc* 1994;69:409–15.

23. Svaninger G, Nordgren S, Oresland T, et al. Incidence and characteristics of pouchitis in the Kock continent ileostomy and the IPAA. *Scand J Gastroenterol* 1993;28:695–700.

24. Sandborn WJ, McLeod R, Jewell DP. Medical therapy for induction and maintenance of remission in pouchitis: a systematic review. *Inflamm Bowel Dis* 1999;5:33–9.

25. Gionchetti P, Rizzello F, Helwig U, et al. Prophylaxis of pouchitis onset with probiotic therapy: a double blind, placebo controlled trial. *Gastroenterology* 2003;124:1202–9.

26. Gionchetti P, Rizzello F, Venturi A, et al. Maintenance treatment of chronic pouchitis: a randomised placebo-controlled double-blind trial with a new probiotic preparation. *Gastroenterology* 1998;114:A985.

27. Stern H, Walfisch S, Mullen B, et al. Cancer in an ileoanal reservoir: a new late complication? *Gut* 1990;4:473–5.

28. Puthu D, Rajan N, Rao R, et al. Carcinoma of the rectal pouch following restorative proctocolectomy. *Dis Colon Rectum* 1992;35:257–60.

29. Rodriguez-Sanjuan JC, Polavieja MG, Naranjo A, et al. Adenocarcinoma in an ileal pouch for ulcerative colitis. *Dis Colon Rectum* 1995;38:779–80.

30. Sequens R. Cancer in the anal canal (transitional zone) after restorative proctocolectomy with stapled ileal-pouch anastomosis. *Int J Colorectal Dis* 1997;1´.:254–5.

31. Rotholtz NA, Pikarsky AJ, Singh JJ, et al. Adenocarcinoma arising from along the rectal stump after double-stapled ileorectal J-pouch in a patient with ulcerative colitis: the need to perform a distal anastomosis. Report of a case. *Dis Colon Rectum* 2001;44:1214–17.

32. Baratsis S, Hadjidimitriou F, Christodoulou M, et al. Adenocarcinoma in the anal canal after ileal pouch-anal anastomosis for ulcerative colitis using a double stapling technique: report of a case. *Dis Colon Rectum* 2002;45:687–91; discussion 691–2.

33. Laureti S, Ugolini F, D'Errico A, et al. Adenocarcinoma below ileoanal anastomosis for ulcerative colitis: report of a case and review of the literature. *Dis Colon Rectum* 2002;45:418–21.

34. Negi SS, Chaudhary A, Gondal R. Carcinoma of IPAA following restorative proctocolectomy: report of a case and review of the literature. *Dig Surg* 2003;20:63–5.

35. Hyman N. Rectal cancer as a complication of stapled IPAA. *Inflamm Bowel Dis* 2002;8:43–5.

36. Veress B, Reinholt FP, Lindquist K, et al. Long-term histomorphological surveillance of the pelvic ileal pouch: dysplasia develops in a subgroup of patients. *Gastroenterology* 1995;109:1090–7.

37. Vieth M, Grunewald M, Niemeyer C, et al. Adenocarcinoma in an ileal pouch after prior proctocolectomy for carcinoma in a patient with ulcerative pancolitis. *Virchows Arch* 1998;433:281–4.

38. Iwama T, Kamikawa J, Higuchi T, et al. Development of invasive adenocarcinoma in a long-standing diverted ileal J-pouch for ulcerative colitis: report of a case. *Dis Colon Rectum* 2000;43:101–4.

39. Heuschen UA, Heuschen G, Autschbach F, et al. Adenocarcinoma in the ileal pouch: late risk of cancer after restorative proctocolectomy. *Int J Colorectal Dis* 2001;16:126–30.

40. Hassan C, Zullo A, Speziale G, et al. Adenocarcinoma of the ileoanal pouch anastomosis: an emerging complication? *Int J Colorectal Dis* 2003;18:276–8.

41. Thompson-Fawcett MW, Marcus V, Redston M, et al. Risk of dysplasia in long-term ileal pouches and pouches with chronic pouchitis. *Gastroenterology* 2001;121:275–81.

42. Lofberg R, Brostrom O, Karlen P, et al. DNA aneuploidy in ulcerative colitis: reproducibility, topographic distribution, and relation to dysplasia. *Gastroenterology* 1992;102:1149–54.

43. Ording Olsen K, Juul S, Berndtsson I, et al. Ulcerative colitis: female fecundity before diagnosis, during disease, and after surgery compared with a population sample. *Gastroenterology* 2002;122:15–19.

44. Ravid A, Richard CS, Spencer LM, et al. Pregnancy, delivery, and pouch function after ileal pouch-anal anastomosis for ulcerative colitis. *Dis Colon Rectum* 2002;45:1283–8.

45. Hahnloser D, Pemberton JH, Wolff BG, et al. Pregnancy and delivery after ileal pouch-anal anastomosis (IPAA) for inflammatory bowel diseases: immediate and long-term consequences and outcomes. Presented at the ASCRS Annual Meeting, June 2003.

46. McLeod RS, Churchill DN, Lock AM, et al. Quality of life of patients with ulcerative colitis preoperatively and postoperatively. *Gastroenterology* 1991;101:1307–13.

47. Jimmo B, Hyman NH. Is ileal pouch-anal anastomosis really the procedure of choice for patients with ulcerative colitis? *Dis Colon Rectum* 1998;41:41–5.

48. Provenzale D, Shearin M, Phillips-Bute B, et al. Health-related quality of life after ileoanal pull-through evaluation and assessment of new health status measures. *Gastroenterology* 1997;113:7–14.

49. Doemeny JM, Burke DR, Meranze SG. Percutaneous drainage of abscesses in patients with Crohn's disease. *Gastrointest Radiol* 1988;13:237–41.

50. Gervais DA, Hahn PF, O'Neill MJ, et al. Percutaneous abscess drainage in Crohn disease: technical success and short- and long-term outcomes during 14 years. *Radiology* 2002;222:645–51.

51. Brown CJ, Buie WD. Perioperative stress dose steroids: do they make a difference? *J Am Coll Surg* 2001;193:678–86.

52. Brezezinski A, Armstrong A, Del Real GA, et al. Infliximab does not increase the risk of complications in the perioperative period in patients with Crohn's disease. *Gastroenterology* 2002;122:A617.

53. Poulin EC, Schlachta CM, Mamazza J, et al. Should enteric fistulas from Crohn's disease or diverticulitis be treated laparoscopically or by open surgery? A matched cohort study. *Dis Colon Rectum* 2000;43:621–6; discussion 626–7.

54. Evans J, Poritz L, MacRae HM. Influence of experience on laparoscopic ileocolic resection for Crohn's disease. *Dis Colon Rectum* 2002;45:1595–600.

55. Schmidt CM, Talamini MA, Kaufman HS, et al. Laparoscopic surgery for Crohn's disease: reasons for conversion. *Ann Surg* 2001;233:733–9.

56. Duepree HJ, Senagore AJ, Delaney CP, et al. Advantages of laparoscopic resection for ileocecal Crohn's disease. *Dis Colon Rectum* 2002;45:605–10.

57. Tabet J, Hong D, Kim CW, et al. Laparoscopic versus open bowel resection for Crohn's disease. *Can J Gastroenterol* 2001;15:237–42.

58. Young-Fadok TM, HallLong K, McConnell EJ, et al. Advantages of laparoscopic resection for ileocolic Crohn's disease. Improved outcomes and reduced costs. *Surg Endosc* 2001;15:450–4.

59. Milsom JW, Hammerhofer KA, Bohm B, et al. Prospective, randomized trial comparing laparoscopic vs conventional surgery for refractory ileocolic Crohn's disease. *Dis Colon Rectum* 2001;44:1–8; discussion 8–9.

60. McLeod RS. Resection margins and recurrent Crohn's disease. *Hepatogastroenterology* 1990;37:63–6.
61. Rutgeerts P, Geboes K, Vantrappen G, et al. Natural history of recurrent Crohn's disease at the ileocolonic anastomosis after curative surgery. *Gut* 1984;25:665–72.
62. Olaison G, Smedh K, Sjodahl R. Natural course of Crohn's disease after ileocolic resection: endoscopically visualized ileal ulcers preceding symptoms. *Gut* 1992;33:331–5.
63. McLeod RS, Wolff BG, Steinhart AH, et al. Risk and significance of endoscopic radiological evidence of recurrent Crohn's disease. *Gastroenterology* 1997;113:1823–7.
64. Bernell O, Lapidus A, Hellers G. Risk factors for surgery and recurrence in 907 patients with primary ileocaecal Crohn's disease. *Br J Surg* 2000;87:1697–701.
65. Wolff BG. Factors determining recurrence following surgery for Crohn's disease. *World J Surg* 1998;22:364–9.
66. Fazio VW, Marchetti F, Church M, et al. Effect of resection margins on the recurrence of Crohn's disease in the small bowel. A randomized controlled trial. *Ann Surg* 1996;224:563–71; discussion 571–3.
67. Cameron JL, Hamilton SR, Coleman J, et al. Patterns of ileal recurrence in Crohn's disease. A prospective randomized study. *Ann Surg* 1992;215:546–51; discussion 551–2.
68. Ikeuchi H, Kusunoki M, Yamamura T. Long-term results of stapled and hand-sewn anastomoses in patients with Crohn's disease. *Dig Surg* 2000;17:493–6.
69. Munoz-Juarez M, Yamamoto T, Wolff BG, et al. Wide-lumen stapled anastomosis versus conventional end-to-end anastomosis in the treatment of Crohn's disease. *Dis Colon Rectum* 2001;44:20–5; discussion 25–6.
70. Hashemi M, Novell JR, Lewis AA. Side-to-side stapled anastomosis may delay recurrence in Crohn's disease. *Dis Colon Rectum* 1998;41:1293–6.
71. Kusunoki M, Ikeuchi H, Yanagi H, et al. A comparison of stapled and hand-sewn anastomosis in Crohn's disease. *Dig Surg* 1998;15:679–82.
72. Scott NA, Sue-Ling HM, Hughes LE. Anastomotic configuration does not affect recurrence of Crohn's disease after ileocolonic resection. *Int J Colorectal Dis* 1995;10:67–9.
73. Moskovitz D, McLeod RS, Greenberg GR, et al. Operative and environmental risk factors for recurrence of Crohn's disease. *Int J Colorectal Dis* 1999;14:224–6.
74. Lee EC, Papaioannou N. Minimal surgery for chronic obstruction in patients with extensive or universal Crohn's disease. *Ann R Coll Surg Engl* 1982;64:229–33.
75. Michelassi F, Hurst RD, Melis M, et al. Side-to-side isoperistaltic strictureplasty in extensive Crohn's disease: a prospective longitudinal study. *Ann Surg* 2000;232:401–8.
76. Poggioli G, Stocchi L, Laureti S, et al. Conservative surgical management of terminal ileitis side-to-side enterocolic anastomosis. *Dis Colon Rectum* 1997;40:234–7; discussion 238–9.
77. Tichansky D, Cagir B, Yoo E, et al. Strictureplasty for Crohn's disease: meta-analysis. *Dis Colon Rectum* 2000;43:911–19.
78. Dietz DW, Laureti S, Strong SA, et al. Safety and longterm efficacy of strictureplasty in 314 patients with obstructing small bowel Crohn's disease. *J Am Coll Surg* 2001;192:330–7; discussion 337–8.
79. Hurst RD, Michelassi F. Strictureplasty for Crohn's disease: techniques and long-term results. *World J Surg* 1998;22:359–63.
80. Borley NR, Mortensen NJ, Chaudry MA, et al. Recurrence after abdominal surgery for Crohn's disease: relationship to disease site and surgical procedure. *Dis Colon Rectum* 2002;45:377–83.
81. Andrews HA, Lewis P, Allan RN. Prognosis after surgery for colonic Crohn's disease. *Br J Surg* 1989;76:1184–90.

82. Farmer RG, Hawk WA, Turnbull RB Jr. Indications for surgery in Crohn's disease: analysis of 500 cases. *Gastroenterology* 1976;71:245–50.
83. Andersson P, Olaison G, Bodemar G, et al. Surgery for Crohn colitis over a twenty-eight year period: fewer stomas and the replacement of total colectomy by segmental resection. *Scand J Gastroenterol* 2002;37:68–73.
84. Longo WE, Oakley JR, Lavery IC, et al. Outcome of ileorectal anastomosis for Crohn's colitis. *Dis Colon Rectum* 1992;35:1066–71.
85 Regimbeau JM, Panis Y, Pocard M, et al. Long-term results of ileal pouch-anal anastomosis for colorectal Crohn's disease. *Dis Colon Rectum* 2001;44:769–78.
86. Hyman NH, Fazio VW, Tuckson WB, et al. Consequences of ileal pouch-anal anastomosis for Crohn's colitis. *Dis Colon Rectum* 1991;34:653–7.
87. Grobler SP, Hosie KB, Affie E, et al. Outcome of restorative proctocolectomy when the diagnosis is suggestive of Crohn's disease. *Gut* 1993;34:1384–8.
88. Peyregne V, Francois Y, Gilly FN, et al. Outcome of ileal pouch after secondary diagnosis of Crohn's disease. *Int J Colorectal Dis* 2000;15:49–53.
89. Yu CS, Pemberton JH, Larson D. Ileal pouch-anal anastomosis in patients with indeterminate colitis: long term results. *Dis Colon Rectum* 2000;43:1487–96.
90. Atkinson KG, Owen DA, Wankling G. Restorative proctocolectomy and indeterminate colitis. *Am J Surg* 1994;167:516–18.
91. Koltun WA, Schoetz DJ Jr, Roberts PL, et al. Indeterminate colitis predisposes to perineal complications after ileal pouch-anal anastomosis. *Dis Colon Rectum* 1991;34:857–60.
92. Buchmann P, Alexander-Williams J. Classification of perianal Crohn's disease. *Clin Gastroenterol* 1980;9:323–30.
93. Van Outryve MJ, Pelckmans PA, Michielsen PP, et al. Value of transrectal ultrasonography in Crohn's disease. *Gastroenterology* 1991;101:1171–7.
94. Solomon MJ, McLeod RS, Cohen EK, et al. Anal wall thickness under normal and inflammatory conditions of the anorectum as determined by endoluminal ultrasonography. *Am J Gastroenterol* 1995;90:574–8.
95. Haggett PJ, Moore NR, Shearman JD, et al. Pelvic and perineal complications of Crohn's disease: assessment using magnetic resonance imaging. *Gut* 1995;36:407–10.
96. Jenss H, Starlinger M, Skaleij M. Magnetic resonance imaging in perianal Crohn's disease. *Lancet* 1992;340:1286.
97. Lunniss PJ, Barker PG, Sultan AH, et al. Magnetic resonance imaging of fistula-in-ano. *Dis Colon Rectum* 1994;37:708–18.
98. Williams JG, MacLeod CA, Rothenberger DA, et al. Seton treatment of high anal fistulae. *Br J Surg* 1991;78:1159–61.
99. Matos D, Lunniss PJ, Phillips RK. Total sphincter conservation in high fistula in ano: results of a new approach. *Br J Surg* 1993;80:802–4.
100. Winter AM, Banks PA, Petros JG. Healing of transsphincteric perianal fistulas in Crohn's disease using a new technique. *Am J Gastroenterol* 1993;88:2022–5.
101. Present DH, Rutgeerts P, Targan S, et al. Infliximab for the treatment of fistulas in patients with Crohn's disease. *N Engl J Med* 1999;340:1398–405.
102. van Bodegraven AA, Sloots CE, Felt-Bersma RJ, et al. Endosonographic evidence of persistence of Crohn's disease-associated fistulas after infliximab treatment, irrespective of clinical response. *Dis Colon Rectum* 2002;45:39–45; discussion 45–6.
103. Poritz LS, Rowe WA, Koltun WA. Remicade does not abolish the need for surgery in fistulizing Crohn's disease. *Dis Colon Rectum* 2002;45:771–5.
104. Hull TL, Fazio VW. Surgical approaches to low anovaginal fistula in Crohn's disease. *Am J Surg* 1997;173:95–8.

5

Cancer in IBD patients

Steven H Itzkowitz

Introduction

Patients with longstanding inflammatory bowel disease (IBD) are at increased risk for developing cancers of the gastrointestinal (GI) tract. Indeed, even years after their disease has been controlled with medications, IBD patients still live with the fear of developing cancer. Colorectal cancer (CRC) is the most common cancer in IBD patients. To date, our understanding of CRC pathobiology has come more from studies of patients with ulcerative colitis (UC) than from those with Crohn's disease (CD). This chapter will focus mainly on the problem of CRC, and then address other cancers such as small bowel adenocarcinoma, cholangiocarcinoma, and hematologic malignancies.

Colorectal cancer in IBD patients

Prevalence and incidence of CRC

Based on a meta-analysis of 116 studies from around the world, the prevalence of CRC in patients with UC is approximately 3.7% overall and 5.4% for those with pancolitis [1]. The incidence rate of CRC is approximately 3 per 1,000 person-years duration, with the highest rates in the US and UK [1]. Since 1955, the overall number of cases of CRC in UC patients has increased. A population-based study in Manitoba, Canada, found that the risk for colon cancer among patients with UC or CD is approximately 2- to 3-fold greater than in the general population, and that the risk of rectal cancer is increased 2-fold in UC, but not in CD [2]. The earlier notion that CD patients have a lower risk of CRC than UC patients was derived from studies that included patients with ileitis and studies that did not take into account the extent of colon involved or disease duration, thereby diluting the CRC risk. In fact, when patients with longstanding, anatomically substantial CD are considered, the risk of CRC is similar between CD and UC [3].

CRC risk factors

Several factors that either increase or decrease CRC risk in the setting of IBD have been identified (see **Table 1**).

Duration of colitis

With respect to increasing CRC risk, the most important factor, which has been reproducibly found in many studies, is the duration of colitis. CRC is rarely encountered before 7 years of colitis. Thereafter the risk rises: a UC patient has a cumulative risk for CRC of 2% after 10 years of colitis, 8% after 20 years, and 18% after 30 years [1].

Extent of colitis

The extent of colitis also contributes to higher risk: the more colonic surface that is involved with colitis, the greater the CRC risk. A population-based study of over 3,000 UC patients in Sweden who were examined by barium enema demonstrated an increasing gradient of risk for patients with proctitis (standardized incidence ratio [SIR] 1.7, 95% confidence interval [CI] 0.8–3.2), left-sided colitis (SIR 2.8, 95% CI 1.6–4.4), and pancolitis (SIR 14.8, 95% CI 11.4–18.9) [4]. The trend of increasing CRC risk with greater colonic involvement has been reproducibly observed, regardless of whether the extent of colitis is determined using barium enema or colonoscopic appearance. Backwash ileitis, which reflects perhaps the greatest disease extent, has been correlated with an increased risk of CRC [5].

Increased CRC risk	Decreased CRC risk
Longer duration of colitis	Prophylactic total proctocolectomy
Greater extent of colonic involvement	Surveillance program
Backwash ileitis (possibly)	• regular doctor visits
Family history of CRC	• surveillance colonoscopy
Primary sclerosing cholangitis	• chemoprevention
Young age of IBD onset (some studies)	
Severity of inflammation (possibly)	

Table 1. Factors associated with risk of colorectal cancer (CRC) in inflammatory bowel disease (IBD) patients.

Very few studies have correlated CRC risk with histologic extent of disease, even though microscopic evidence of colitis is arguably a better indicator of disease extent than either endoscopic or radiographic changes. A recent review of 30 colectomy specimens found that dysplasia and CRC can arise in areas of microscopic colitis that are proximal to areas of gross colitis, suggesting that histologic changes, even without colonoscopic alterations, might indeed better define disease extent for the purposes of cancer risk [6].

Family history
IBD patients with a family history of CRC have been reported to have at least a 2-fold higher risk of CRC than IBD patients with no family history of CRC [7–9].

Primary sclerosing cholangitis
The small subset of IBD patients with primary sclerosing cholangitis (PSC) are at particularly high risk for developing CRC [10]. In a population-based Swedish study, the cumulative incidence of CRC in UC patients with PSC was 33% at 20 years [11]. Since the colitis in PSC patients is often asymptomatic, the physician may not consider an evaluation of the colon. Even if colonoscopy does detect underlying colitis, it is hard to know the

precise duration of the colitis. It is therefore important to perform an initial colonoscopy with comprehensive biopsies on any patient with PSC, even in the absence of colonic symptoms.

Young age of IBD onset
Onset of colitis in childhood has been reported to be an independent risk factor for CRC in some [1,4,12], but not all, studies [13,14]. Regardless of these discrepant reports, since younger IBD patients will typically have their disease for longer, they warrant heightened vigilance.

Severity of inflammation
The degree of colitis activity has not been considered an independent risk factor for CRC, but it depends on how disease activity is defined. For example, when disease activity is measured according to the frequency of clinical exacerbations, there does not appear to be a correlation with CRC risk [9]. However, a recent case-control study from St Mark's Hospital, UK, found that histologic evidence of active inflammation was indeed an independent risk factor for CRC [15]. It is important to bear in mind that the patient with quiescent IBD is also at increased CRC risk because they have been able to avoid colectomy for severely active colitis and therefore keep their colon for a longer duration.

Reducing CRC risk

With regard to reducing CRC risk, there are two main choices: remove the colon or conduct a lifelong program of surveillance (see **Table 1**). Clearly, removing the colon and rectum, for example after 7–10 years of colitis, is the ultimate means of preventing CRC. While prophylactic total proctocolectomy is considered quite radical, it may not be unreasonable, especially in young patients who otherwise face several decades of frequent colonoscopic surveillance that still does not guarantee absolute protection against mortality from CRC.

Most patients prefer to keep their colon (assuming it does not have to be otherwise removed because of intractable colitis symptoms), and they are therefore advised to undergo periodic surveillance. Surveillance should be viewed as a program that includes regular visits to the doctor, the use of medications to control inflammation (some of which may have chemopreventive effects, see below), and regular colonoscopies. The goal of surveillance colonoscopy is to detect neoplastic lesions before they become biologically dangerous. Thus, the detection and interpretation of dysplasia is crucial to successful surveillance.

Diagnosing dysplasia

Macroscopic classification

Despite considerable heterogeneity in appearance [16], dysplasia in IBD is often classified macroscopically as raised or flat, depending on whether it corresponds to an endoscopically visible lesion. Raised lesions, conventionally referred to by the term DALM (dysplasia-associated lesion or mass) [17], can appear as polyps, bumps, plaques, and velvety patches [17,18]. Such lesions can blend easily with the gross inflammatory abnormalities that are commonly encountered in IBD colons, making their endoscopic detection difficult, even for experienced practitioners.

Flat dysplasia is detected microscopically in random biopsies from unremarkable mucosa. Its detection therefore depends on adequate sampling of the mucosa by the endoscopist. Rubin et al. calculated that 33 and 64 biopsies are required to detect dysplasia with 90% and 95% probability, respectively [19]. Current practice guidelines recommend that 2–4 biopsies are taken from every 10 cm of diseased colon, in addition to macroscopically atypical lesions [20]; however, since <0.05% of the total colonic surface area is thereby sampled, even rigid adherence to these guidelines will not eliminate false-negative examinations. Indeed, results from questionnaire surveys have suggested that the number of biopsies taken by endoscopists in routine practice often falls short of recommended guidelines [21,22].

The significance of dysplasia in endoscopically visible lesions came from studies that reported high rates of cancer when patients with such lesions underwent colectomy [17,18]. Blackstone et al. reported cancers in seven of 12 DALM-bearing colons, including five with only mild or moderate dysplasia in preoperative biopsies [17]. A subsequent compilation of published results from 10 surveillance programs reported cancers in 17 of 40 (43%) colectomies performed because of DALM [23]. It was concluded that DALM is an indication for colectomy, irrespective of the grade of dysplasia in preoperative biopsies. While not fully appreciated at the time, the original studies of DALM dealt exclusively with lesions that could not be removed endoscopically for microscopic examination. Thus, the significance of such lesions as an indication for surgery is similar to that of endoscopically nonresectable sporadic adenomatous polyps, which frequently harbor invasive cancer at the polyp base despite the presence of low-grade dysplasia (LGD) in their more biopsy-accessible upper portions.

Significance of dysplasia
More recently, we have come to realize that not all types of polypoid dysplasia in patients with IBD carry the same significance. Some polyps may be adenomatous polyps unrelated to colitis that can be managed by endoscopic polypectomy in the same manner as polyps in the general population [24–26]. One example is the dysplastic polyp encountered in a bowel segment that is entirely free of disease (eg, in the proximal colon of a patient with left-sided UC). In such cases, one would take the precaution to biopsy the mucosa surrounding the polyp to assure the absence of microscopic disease. Similarly, a dysplastic polyp with a well-defined stalk can be regarded as a sporadic adenoma, even when encountered in a colitic region, if the mucosa lining its stalk is nondysplastic.

Conservative management is also reasonable for dysplastic polyps that are "adenoma-like" [27,28]. These polyps are endoscopically indistinguishable from sporadic sessile adenomatous polyps – ie, they are discrete, ovoid or round, completely resectable by the endoscope, and not surrounded by flat dysplasia. Such lesions have long posed a dilemma for endoscopists who are familiar with the DALM concept, but are reluctant to advocate colectomy for what appear to be innocuous lesions and possibly nothing more than adenomas. Histology has not provided a reliable means of making this distinction in individual cases [29], since the histologic features of dysplasia can be virtually identical in the setting of IBD and in true adenomas. A 1999 study from the Mount Sinai Hospital in New York reported that conservative management of a cohort of 48 UC patients with a total of 70 such polyps, including three with high-grade dysplasia (HGD), resulted in no adverse outcomes during a mean follow-up period of 4.1 years [27]. Similar conclusions were reached in a concurrent study from the Brigham and Women's Hospital, Boston [28]. As a result, the burden of deciding whether a polyp qualifies as adenoma-like rests with the endoscopist. Molecular markers may ultimately afford a more objective means of making these distinctions [30,31], but, as yet, these analyses are not applicable to routine clinical practice.

Microscopic classification

GI dysplasia is defined microscopically as replacement of the native intestinal epithelium by an unequivocally neoplastic, but noninvasive, epithelium [32]. It is synonymous with the term "intraepithelial neoplasia" used in other organ systems. The histologic classification of dysplasia in IBD is based on Riddell and colleagues' 1983 consensus report, in which a group of expert GI pathologists proposed classifying biopsies into five categories [32]:

- negative for dysplasia

- indefinite for dysplasia

- LGD

- HGD

- invasive cancer

Although they recommended a further subdivision of the indefinite category (into probably negative, probably positive, and unknown), many pathologists regard this as optional.

The cellular abnormalities that define dysplasia in IBD are analogous to those that characterize neoplastic tissue in general, namely nuclear abnormalities reflecting inappropriate cellular proliferation and cytoplasmic abnormalities reflecting clonality and aberrant differentiation. The distinction between LGD and HGD depends upon the distribution of nuclei within the cells: LGD is characterized by nuclei that remain confined to the basal half of the cells, and HGD by nuclei that are stratified haphazardly between the basal and apical halves [32]. Not surprisingly, pathologists are frequently confronted with biopsies that lie in a gray zone between the two categories, and some degree of subjectivity is therefore unavoidable. The diagnostic category "indefinite for dysplasia" is an acknowledgment of the great difficulty that pathologists face in discriminating between dysplasia and reactive epithelial changes, although experienced pathologists are usually able to differentiate between the two.

Most studies comparing diagnoses of dysplasia among different pathologists, both prospectively and retrospectively, have concluded that levels of interobserver agreement are fair at best, even among specialists in GI pathology [33–38]. The best agreement levels tend to occur at the two extremes of negative and HGD, and the poorest levels in the gray zone between LGD and HGD and the gray zones on either side of indefinite for dysplasia. From a practical standpoint, it has been recommended that diagnoses carrying serious management implications be reviewed by at least one additional pathologist with expertise in this area [32].

Biology of dysplasia

Natural history

The natural history of dysplasia is a key factor that contributes to the outcome and success of surveillance. A convenient paradigm proposes that colon carcinogenesis in IBD follows a progression from no dysplasia to indefinite dysplasia, LGD, HGD, and, finally, invasive cancer. While this model is conceptually useful, it is by no means absolute. There are instances in which patients undergoing regular colonoscopic surveillance have developed CRC without any prior dysplasia. Likewise, it is not necessary for LGD to progress to HGD before cancer arises in the colon [16,39]. This highlights the need to develop markers that are complementary to dysplasia for predicting CRC risk in IBD patients – a subject of ongoing investigation.

In the meantime, we currently rely upon the histologic identification of dysplasia to make management decisions. Refinements in interpreting dysplasia based on the 1983 standardized histologic criteria [32] have enabled a more accurate prediction of which patients are more likely to progress to advanced neoplasia by excluding those whose biopsies only show reactive changes secondary to inflammation. This was amply illustrated by the St Mark's group, who found that the 5-year cumulative rate of progression from LGD to HGD or invasive cancer rose from 16% to 54% once biopsies were more precisely reclassified [37,40].

When considering the natural history of dysplasia, it is important to bear in mind that patients may already have CRC at the time dysplasia is discovered. A review of 10 prospective surveillance trials published before 1994 found that 42% (10/24) of patients with HGD and 16% (3/19) of patients with LGD who underwent immediate colectomy had synchronous CRC [23]. Likewise, a more recent study from the Mount Sinai Hospital found that 27% (3/11) of patients who underwent colectomy within 6 months of the initial detection of flat LGD had a surprise finding of cancer or HGD [39].

Progression
Assuming that early colectomy is not performed, what is the subsequent rate of progression? In the case of patients with

HGD, 32% were found to have CRC after some follow-up period; for those with LGD, the probability of eventually progressing to HGD or CRC was 16%–29% [23]. Data from St Mark's Hospital indicate that the 5-year cumulative probability of progressing from LGD to HGD or cancer is 54% [37]. Strikingly similar results were obtained from the Mount Sinai Hospital, with a 5-year progression rate of 53% among 46 patients with initial flat LGD [39]. Likewise, a series of 18 patients with LGD followed at the Mayo Clinic demonstrated a 33% 5-year progression rate [41].

In contrast to these studies, other authors have reported substantially lower rates of progression. A series from the Karolinska Institute, Sweden, observed that among 60 patients with LGD, there was no progression to cancer and only two cases of progression to HGD in DALM over a mean follow-up period of 10 years [42]. A group from Leeds, UK, demonstrated that only 10% (3/29) of patients with LGD progressed to HGD or cancer after 10 years [43]. It is worth noting that the designation of LGD in the latter two studies included specimens that were interpreted prior to the 1983 consensus guidelines, and might therefore have included cases of indefinite dysplasia.

Whether these disparate findings are due to differences in patient populations, pathologic interpretation, or other factors, the decision to tie the patient's future to either the 0%–10% or the 33%–54% rate of progression of LGD has to be made by both the clinician and the patient. To assist with their decision making, some physicians recommend colectomy only if LGD is repeatedly confirmed on follow-up examinations, or in more than one specimen per examination ("multifocal LGD"). However, this is a risky strategy. First, a negative examination following one in which LGD was found does not offer reassurance that the patient's risk has declined; the vast majority of such patients will eventually have LGD or an even worse pathology on subsequent colonoscopies or colectomy [39,44]. Second, recent work from my group indicates that the rate of progression of unifocal LGD is essentially identical to that of multifocal LGD [39]. Therefore, once flat LGD is detected in a colitic colon, even in a focal area (assuming it is confirmed by an expert GI pathologist), the patient is at heightened risk of developing CRC and early colectomy should be strongly considered.

Management of dysplasia
Once the decision is made to place a patient under surveillance, it is recommended that the patient formally agree to enter such a program and is willing to comply with it. Patients must be made to understand the limitations of surveillance and accept that, despite their own cooperation, dysplasia and cancer can still arise, even if they are in the hands of skilled endoscopists and pathologists [37].

The best proof that surveillance colonoscopy effectively reduces CRC mortality would be a prospective randomized controlled trial in which patients with longstanding IBD would undergo colonoscopic surveillance while controls matched for a similar risk profile would not. However, due to ethical, financial, and practical limitations, this type of study will probably never come to pass. We must therefore rely on retrospective studies for insights as to the efficacy of surveillance colonoscopy. So far, the best evidence that colonoscopy reduces mortality from CRC in UC comes from case-control studies. In one such study, CRC mortality was reduced by as much as 78%, although this study lacked statistical power [45]. Another investigation found a similar degree of protection [9]. In these studies, a protective effect was found for individuals who had just one or two surveillance examinations. There is also good evidence from prospective (albeit uncontrolled) studies of surveillance colonoscopy that, in general, patients who comply with surveillance have cancers detected at an earlier stage compared with those who do not comply [37,46]. Of course, cancers will still arise even within a surveillance program, but, on balance, the practice of surveillance is beneficial [47].

Although the gastroenterology community has put its faith in surveillance colonoscopy to prevent mortality from CRC in IBD patients, surveillance has its drawbacks. The considerable interobserver disagreement that exists between general pathologists and GI pathologists, and even among expert GI pathologists themselves, has been mentioned above. Endoscopists also have difficulty in recognizing dysplasia. Unlike the dysplastic sporadic adenoma that typically assumes a discrete, polypoid shape surrounded by normal mucosa, dysplasia in the colitic colon can be flat or polypoid and is often difficult to discern. This may be particularly troublesome in a colon that is replete with inflammatory pseudopolyps. The fact that endoscopists do not always take a sufficient number of biopsies of the colon during surveillance examinations contributes to problems of endoscopic detection.

There is also poor understanding of dysplasia amongst trained gastroenterologists. In a survey of practicing gastroenterologists and senior GI fellows in the US, only 19% of respondents correctly identified dysplasia as neoplastic change [21]. Patient compliance is another factor that must be considered when measuring the success of a surveillance program. Patient drop-out or noncompliance with surveillance makes an important contribution to CRC mortality in IBD [37,43] and this must be considered when embarking upon, or continuing, a course of surveillance in individual patients.

Recommended surveillance strategy

Patients with UC
Despite the limitations of surveillance colonoscopy, dysplasia remains the best marker for managing cancer risk in IBD. Based on the natural history of dysplasia discussed above, I propose the following surveillance strategy (see **Figure 1**). After approximately 7–8 years of colitis, patients should undergo an "initial" surveillance colonoscopy to determine the extent of colitis and check for neoplasia. The entire colon should be

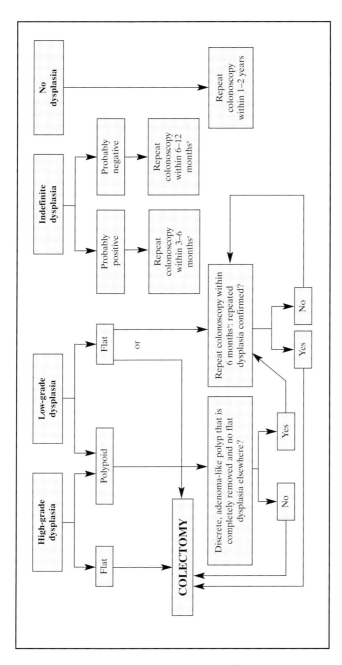

Figure 1. Suggested surveillance strategy for cancer in inflammatory bowel disease patients. [a]Duration of short-term surveillance has not been determined.

examined, with approximately four biopsies taken every 10 cm. Some experts suggest taking more biopsies in the distal rectosigmoid (eg, approximately every 5 cm) since the distribution of neoplasia in UC shows a distal predominance. Biopsies should be taken from flat mucosa, and any suspicious lesions that are encountered should be removed if possible and processed in separate specimen containers (with additional biopsies taken near the base of the polyp). If a patient is experiencing moderate to severe colitis symptoms, it is prudent to control the inflammation medically prior to the examination in order to minimize difficulties with the histologic interpretation of dysplasia. Nonetheless, active inflammation should not preclude the interpretation of dysplasia by expert pathologists and is no reason to refrain from performing surveillance biopsies.

If no dysplasia is detected, the examination should be repeated in 1–2 years. This interval is derived, in part, from studies reporting that interval cancers can develop within 2 years of a surveillance examination [37]. If indefinite dysplasia is reported, the nature of the uncertainty should be discussed with the pathologist. If the suspicion of dysplasia is high (ie, probably positive), a repeat biopsy may be indicated within 3–6 months or less; if suspicion is low, the interval can be lengthened to every 6–12 months. If LGD is detected in a discrete polyp that can be readily resected endoscopically and there is no flat dysplasia immediately adjacent to the polyp or elsewhere in the colon, surveillance can be continued, although the frequency of examinations can be temporarily reduced to every 3–6 months, particularly to re-evaluate the area of polypectomy. Tattoo of the polypectomy site is advised to permit relocalization of the area on subsequent examinations.

If LGD is detected in flat mucosa (whether unifocal or multifocal) and is confirmed by a second expert GI pathologist, colectomy should be strongly considered. If the patient refuses colectomy, repeat surveillance examinations should be undertaken within 3–6 months or less. However, the patient should be advised that a negative subsequent examination is no assurance of safety, and that temporizing until there is histologic progression to HGD or cancer is risky.

A patient in whom flat HGD or adenocarcinoma is confirmed by two expert pathologists should undergo colectomy unless serious comorbidities dictate otherwise. If HGD is diagnosed in an adenoma-like polyp, but is completely removed without evidence of flat dysplasia in the adjacent mucosa or elsewhere in the colon, continued surveillance can be considered. As with any set of recommendations, decisions should be individualized according to the situation of the patient. Hopefully, strategies for surveillance will become more refined as greater knowledge of the natural history of dysplasia is obtained.

Patients with Crohn's colitis

Much less is known with respect to the effectiveness of surveillance in patients with Crohn's colitis. To date, only one practice-based retrospective surveillance study has been reported in patients with Crohn's colitis [48]. Of 259 patients with Crohn's colitis affecting at least one third of the colon for at least 8 years, 16% were found to have dysplasia or cancer over a 16-year period in which 663 examinations were performed, and there were no cancer-related deaths. While we await additional data on the subject, it seems wise to follow a UC-based surveillance strategy for patients with at least 8 years of substantial Crohn's colitis.

An important question that remains to be answered is whether patients with dysplasia or cancer in the setting of segmental Crohn's colitis can undergo segmental resection of the involved area or whether they should proceed to a more extensive, UC-like surgical approach. Another dilemma that is encountered with Crohn's colitis, more so than with UC, is the management of strictures. The finding of a stricture in the colon of a UC patient usually indicates an underlying malignancy, especially if the stricture is causing symptoms and is located in the proximal colon [49]. However, since most strictures in Crohn's colitis are benign, the Crohn's colitis patient can often be managed conservatively. Surveillance of such patients often requires a narrower colonoscope or sometimes dilation of the stricture to visualize the proximal mucosa [48]. Consideration should be given to adding brush cytology of strictures to regular forceps biopsies, and performing a barium enema to evaluate colonic wall irregularity.

Chemoprevention

Despite the relative protection afforded by surveillance colonoscopies in IBD, some patients will still develop CRC. This raises the issue of whether chemoprevention, in the form of either medications or dietary supplements, might help to reduce the risk of CRC in IBD. **Table 2** summarizes the studies in this field.

NSAIDs

With respect to sporadic CRC, it is now well established that aspirin and other nonsteroidal anti-inflammatory drugs (NSAIDs) can significantly reduce the incidence of, and mortality from, CRC. Since many patients with IBD take NSAIDs in the form of 5-aminosalicylates (5-ASA), investigators have asked whether 5-ASA compounds might also be protective. Although no study has yet been undertaken specifically to address this question in a prospective manner, the available data suggest that this may be the case (see **Table 2**). Initial observations by Lashner and colleagues reported a markedly increased risk of colorectal neoplasia in patients who were allergic to sulfa and were therefore not taking sulfasalazine [50]. However, patients who took sulfasalazine did not demonstrate a risk reduction in either this study or in the subsequent cohort study [51]. Further studies that took into account dose and duration of use found a protective role for sulfasalazine when taken for longer than a 3-month period [52] or when taken at doses >2 g/day [9]. In fact, Eaden and coworkers reported a 75% colon cancer risk reduction for individuals taking regular 5-ASA compounds [9]. The risk reduction was greatest for mesalazine compared with other similar compounds, and aspirin use *per se* had no protective effect, although the number of patients taking aspirin was small.

Further support for a protective effect of NSAIDs comes from the study of Bansal and Sonnenberg, who reviewed the Veterans Affairs patient discharge database from 1981–1993 (over 3.41 million discharges) and identified 371 patients with the diagnosis of IBD and CRC [53]. By searching the database for individuals who were also diagnosed with cardiovascular or rheumatologic disorders that would warrant treatment with NSAIDs, they found that IBD patients who also carried NSAID-associated diagnoses had a slight, although not statistically significant, decrease in the risk of developing CRC (odds ratio 0.84), but a statistically significant reduction in death from CRC (odds ratio 0.51). Despite these positive studies, a population-based study found no apparent protective effect of 5-ASA [54]. Likewise, Tung and colleagues found no protective effect of sulfasalazine, but this may be due to the fact that they only included IBD patients with PSC – a highly selected subgroup of IBD patients at particularly high risk for CRC [55].

Steroids
If 5-ASA compounds prevent CRC by suppressing inflammation, it follows that other anti-inflammatory medications used in IBD patients should also be protective against CRC. Although one study reported that the use of systemic steroids and even topical steroids resulted in a significant CRC risk reduction, other studies have been unable to show a similar beneficial effect of steroids or other immunomodulators (see **Table 2**). More research is required to better elucidate this area.

Folate
In the setting of sporadic CRC, low folate intake has been associated with an increased risk for developing colorectal adenomas and carcinomas [56,57]. Patients with chronic IBD are

Reference	Medication	OR or RR	95% CI	P-value
Aminosalicylates/NSAIDs				
Lashner et al., 1989 [50]	Sulfa allergy (no sulfasalazine use)	11.71	1.65–83.10	<0.05
	Sulfasalazine use	1.50	0.43–5.19	NS
Lashner et al., 1997 [51]	Sulfasalazine	0.95	0.34–2.70	NS
	Mesalamine	0.88	0.21–3.73	NS
Pinczowski et al., 1994 [52]	Sulfasalazine:			
	Never or treatment <3 months	–	–	–
	≥1 course >3 months	0.34	0.19–0.62	Significant
Eaden et al., 2000 [9]	5-ASA			
	No	–	–	–
	Yes	0.25	0.13–0.48	<0.00001
	Mesalazine			
	<1.2 g/day	0.08	0.08–0.85	0.04
	>1.2 g/day	0.09	0.03–0.28	<0.00001
	Sulfasalazine			
	<2 g/day	0.56	0.17–1.84	NS
	>2 g/day	0.41	0.18–0.92	0.03
	Olsalazine, balsalazide	0.40	0.04–3.58	NS
	Aspirin (yes, compared to none)	0.80	0.21–2.98	NS
Bansal and Sonnenberg, 1996 [53]	NSAID-associated diagnoses			
	Risk of developing CRC	0.84	0.65–1.08	NS
	Risk of CRC mortality	0.51	0.28–0.94	0.03
Bernstein et al., 2003 [54]	5-ASA	1.46	0.58–3.73	NS
Tung et al., 2001 [55]	Sulfasalazine	3.3	0.8–14	NS
	5-ASA	0.88	0.25–3.20	NS

Reference	Medication	OR or RR	95% CI	P-value
Steroids				
Lashner et al., 1997 [51]	Prednisone	1.52	0.55–4.16	NS
Eaden et al., 2000 [9]	Systemic steroids (yes, compared to none)	0.26	0.01–0.70	0.008
	Local steroids (yes, compared to none)	0.44	0.19–1.02	0.06
Tung et al., 2001 [55]	Prednisone	0.50	0.16–1.5	NS
Immunomodulators				
Lashner et al., 1997 [51]	Azathioprine	1.12	0.26–4.77	NS
Tung et al., 2001 [55]	Azathioprine	0.68	0.17–2.6	NS
	Methotrexate	2.7	0.23–31	NS
	Cyclosporine	0.57	0.15–2.2	NS
Folate				
Lashner et al., 1989 [50]	Folate supplements	0.38	0.12–1.20	NS
Lashner et al., 1997 [51]	Folate	0.72	0.28–1.83	NS
Ursodeoxycholic acid				
Tung et al., 2001 [55]	Ursodiol	0.18	0.05–0.61	0.005
Pardi et al., 2003 [58]	Ursodiol	0.26	0.06–0.99	0.034

Table 2. Colorectal cancer (CRC) risk reduction in inflammatory bowel disease patients related to medication usage. 5-ASA: 5-aminosalicylates; CI: confidence interval; NS: not significant; NSAIDS: nonsteroidal anti-inflammatory drugs; OR: odds ratio; RR: relative risk.

predisposed towards folate deficiency because of inadequate nutritional intake, excessive intestinal losses with active disease, and reduced intestinal absorption due to competitive inhibition from sulfasalazine use. The results of two studies have suggested a trend towards protection against CRC in folate users, although neither study demonstrated statistical significance (see **Table 2**) [50,51]. Nonetheless, since it is safe and inexpensive, folate supplementation should be considered for CRC risk reduction in patients with longstanding IBD.

Ursodiol

In animal models of colon carcinogenesis, ursodiol inhibits carcinogenesis – an effect that may be due to the ursodiol reducing the colonic concentration of the secondary bile acid deoxycholic acid. Ursodiol also has antioxidant activity. A study of UC patients with PSC demonstrated that ursodiol use was strongly associated with a decreased prevalence of colonic dysplasia (see **Table 2**) [55]. This protective effect remained after adjusting for duration of colitis, age at onset of colitis, and sulfasalazine use. Likewise, in a study of PSC patients followed at the Mayo Clinic, ursodiol use was associated with significant protection against the development of dysplasia and cancer [58]. At the present time, however, we do not know whether ursodiol can prevent neoplastic progression in UC patients without PSC.

Other cancers in IBD patients

Small bowel adenocarcinoma

Patients with CD are at increased risk for small bowel adenocarcinoma, especially those with ileitis or ileocolitis. Although the absolute number of cases of small bowel adenocarcinoma is low, this cancer is rare in the general population, leading to a risk that is approximately 10- to 12-fold greater in CD patients than in the general population [2,59]. The symptoms overlap with those of CD, so the diagnosis of small bowel adenocarcinoma is typically made at the time of surgery. Risk factors include long duration of disease and, in some studies, male gender. There is some suggestion that 5-ASA compounds might lower the risk of small bowel adenocarcinoma [59].

Squamous cell carcinoma of the anus

Squamous cell carcinoma of the anus has been reported in patients with longstanding, complicated perianal CD [60]. Worsening perianal symptoms in such patients should warrant heightened vigilance for this tumor, which often requires examination under anesthesia for adequate tissue diagnosis.

Pouch dysplasia

Patients with UC who have undergone total proctocolectomy with ileal pouch-anal anastomosis (IPAA) have a very small risk of dysplasia arising from the ileal mucosa of the pouch itself. The risk is thought to be higher in patients with chronic pouchitis and associated severe villous atrophy [61], but this has not been shown in all series [62]. The risk of dysplasia or cancer is greater in the anal transitional mucosa between the pouch and the anal canal, particularly if a cuff of rectal mucosa has been left, and if the indication for the IPAA was rectal dysplasia or cancer [63]. While there are currently no guidelines for endoscopic surveillance after an IPAA procedure, in those patients who have chronic pouchitis and severe villous atrophy or whose original indication for IPAA was dysplasia or cancer, a program of periodic endoscopy with biopsies is reasonable, paying particular attention to any anal transition zone.

Hepatobiliary cancers

An increased risk for hepatobiliary cancers has been found in UC patients in several [2,64–66], but not all [67], studies. For many of these patients, PSC was the predisposing factor.

Hematologic malignancies

An apparent increase in hematologic malignancies has been reported in patients with UC and CD. Early case series from the Cleveland Clinic [64], the Mount Sinai Hospital [68], and other centers [69] reported an increase in leukemia in patients with UC.

However, population-based studies from Denmark [65], Sweden [67], and Canada [2] have failed to substantiate any increased risk of leukemia. Likewise, although an increased number of lymphomas has been reported in some case series [68,70], other series [64] and several population-based studies [65–67,71] do not support the notion that patients with UC or CD are at increased risk of lymphoma. However, a population-based study from Canada has reported an increased rate of lymphoma among male patients with CD [2]. While there has been some concern that immunomodulatory therapies might predispose patients to lymphoma [72], this concept is based on very few events in case series or anecdotal case reports and has not been confirmed in other case series [73] or population-based studies [2].

Future directions

The future is exciting with respect to new developments in the management of cancer risk in IBD patients. Already, there are reports of using chromoendoscopy with magnifying endoscopes to enhance the detection of dysplasia during colonoscopy. Indeed, chromoendoscopy can increase the yield of dysplasia by 3-fold [74], detecting important lesions that would otherwise go unnoticed.

In the modern era of molecular diagnostics, tissue and even stool samples from patients with IBD can be investigated for molecular alterations. For example, University of Washington investigators have demonstrated that because there is often widespread genomic instability throughout the colon of IBD patients, it may be possible to analyze rectal biopsies by DNA fingerprinting or fluorescence in-situ hybridization methods [75] and identify patients at particularly high risk for cancer. The advent of technology to extract human DNA from stool and look for specific DNA mutations associated with sporadic colon carcinogenesis [76,77] implies that this approach may also be worthwhile in IBD patients. It is anticipated that refinements in our knowledge of cancer biology, clinical practice, and molecular discovery will bring a new level of sophistication to the management of patients with longstanding IBD and lower the incidence of CRC in this high-risk population.

References

1. Eaden J, Abrams KR, Mayberry JF. The risk of colorectal cancer in ulcerative colitis: a meta-analysis. *Gut* 2001;48:526–35.

2. Bernstein CN, Blanchard JF, Kliewer E, et al. Cancer risk in patients with inflammatory bowel disease: a population-based study. *Cancer* 2001;91:854–62.

3. Sachar DB. Cancer in Crohn's disease: dispelling the myths. *Gut* 1994;35:1507–8.

4. Ekbom A, Helmick C, Zack M, et al. Ulcerative colitis and colorectal cancer: a population-based study. *N Engl J Med* 1990;323:1228–33.

5. Heuschen UA, Hinz U, Allemeyer EH, et al. Backwash ileitis is strongly associated with colorectal carcinoma in ulcerative colitis. *Gastroenterology* 2001;120:841–7.

6. Mathy C, Schneider K, Chen YY, et al. Gross versus microscopic pancolitis and the occurrence of neoplasia in ulcerative colitis. *Inflamm Bowel Dis* 2003;9:351–5.

7. Askling J, Dickman PW, Karlen P, et al. Family history as a risk factor for colorectal cancer in inflammatory bowel disease. *Gastroenterology* 2001;120:1356–62.

8. Nuako KW, Ahlquist DA, Mahoney DW, et al. Familial predisposition for colorectal cancer in chronic ulcerative colitis: a case-control study. *Gastroenterology* 1998; 115:1079–83.

9. Eaden J, Abrams K, Ekbom A, et al. Colorectal cancer prevention in ulcerative colitis: a case-control study. *Aliment Pharmacol Ther* 2000;14:145–53.

10. Jayaram H, Satsangi J, Chapman RW. Increased colorectal neoplasia in chronic ulcerative colitis complicated by primary sclerosing cholangitis: fact or fiction? *Gut* 2001;48:430–4.

11. Kornfeld D, Ekbom A, Ihre T. Is there an excess risk for colorectal cancer in patients with ulcerative colitis and concomitant primary sclerosing cholangitis? A population based study. *Gut* 1997;41:522–5.

12. Prior P, Gyde SN, Macartney JC, et al. Cancer morbidity in ulcerative colitis. *Gut* 1982;23:490–7.

13. Greenstein AJ, Sachar DB, Smith H, et al. Cancer in universal and left-sided ulcerative colitis: factors determining risk. *Gastroenterology* 1979;77:290–4.

14. Lennard-Jones JE. Cancer risk in ulcerative colitis: surveillance or surgery. *Br J Surg* 1985;72(Suppl.) S84–6.

15. Rutter M, Saunders B, Wilkinson K, et al. Severity of inflammation is a risk factor for colorectal neoplasia in ulcerative colitis. *Gastroenterology* 2004;126:451–9.

16. Harpaz N, Talbot IC. Colorectal cancer in idiopathic inflammatory bowel disease. *Semin Diagn Pathol* 1996;13:339–57.

17. Blackstone MO, Riddell RH, Rogers BH, et al. Dysplasia-associated lesion or mass (DALM) detected by colonoscopy in long-standing ulcerative colitis: an indication for colectomy. *Gastroenterology* 1981;80:366–74.

18. Butt JH, Konishi F, Morson BC, et al. Macroscopic lesions in dysplasia and carcinoma complicating ulcerative colitis. *Dig Dis Sci* 1983;28:18–26.

19. Rubin CE, Haggitt RC, Burmer GC, et al. DNA aneuploidy in colonic biopsies predicts future development of dysplasia in ulcerative colitis. *Gastroenterology* 1992;103:1611–20.

20. Kornbluth A, Sachar DB. Ulcerative colitis practice guidelines in adults. American College of Gastroenterology, Practice Parameters Committee. *Am J Gastroenterol* 1997;92:204–11.

21. Bernstein CN, Weinstein WM, Levine DS, et al. Physicians' perceptions of dysplasia and approaches to surveillance colonoscopy in ulcerative colitis. *Am J Gastroenterol* 1995;90:2106–14.

22. Eaden JA, Ward BA, Mayberry JF. How gastroenterologists screen for colonic cancer in ulcerative colitis: an analysis of performance. *Gastrointest Endosc* 2000;51:123–8.

23. Bernstein CN, Shanahan F, Weinstein WM. Are we telling patients the truth about surveillance colonoscopy in ulcerative colitis? *Lancet* 1994;343:71–4.

24. Torres C, Antonioli D, Odze RD. Polypoid dysplasia and adenomas in inflammatory bowel disease: a clinical, pathologic, and follow-up study of 89 polyps from 59 patients. *Am J Surg Pathol* 1998;22:275–84.

25. Rozen P, Baratz M, Fefer F, et al. Low incidence of significant dysplasia in a successful endoscopic surveillance program of patients with ulcerative colitis. *Gastroenterology* 1995;108:1361–70.

26. Nugent FW, Haggitt RC, Gilpin PA. Cancer surveillance in ulcerative colitis. *Gastroenterology* 1991;100:1241–8.

27. Rubin PH, Friedman S, Harpaz N, et al. Colonoscopic polypectomy in chronic colitis: conservative management after endoscopic resection of dysplastic polyps. *Gastroenterology* 1999;117:1295–300.

28. Engelsgjerd M, Farraye FA, Odze RD. Polypectomy may be adequate treatment for adenoma-like dysplastic lesions in chronic ulcerative colitis. *Gastroenterology* 1999;117:1288–94; discussion 1488–91.

29. Schneider A, Stolte M. Differential diagnosis of adenomas and dysplastic lesions in patients with ulcerative colitis. *Z Gastroenterol* 1993;31:653–6.

30. Selaru FM, Xu Y, Yin J, et al. Artificial neural networks distinguish among subtypes of neoplastic colorectal lesions. *Gastroenterology* 2002;122:606–13.

31. Odze RD, Brown CA, Hartmann CJ, et al. Genetic alterations in chronic ulcerative colitis-associated adenoma-like DALMs are similar to non-colitic sporadic adenomas. *Am J Surg Pathol* 2000;24:1209–16.

32. Riddell RH, Goldman H, Ransohoff DF, et al. Dysplasia in inflammatory bowel disease: standardized classification with provisional clinical applications. *Hum Pathol* 1983;14:931–68.

33. Eaden J, Abrams K, McKay H, et al. Inter-observer variation between general and specialist gastrointestinal pathologists when grading dysplasia in ulcerative colitis. *J Pathol* 2001;194:152–7.

34. Dixon MF, Brown LJ, Gilmour HM, et al. Observer variation in the assessment of dysplasia in ulcerative colitis. *Histopathology* 1988;13:385–97.

35. Odze RD, Goldblum J, Noffsinger A, et al. Interobserver variability in the diagnosis of ulcerative colitis-associated dysplasia by telepathology. *Mod Pathol* 2002;15:379–86.

36. Melville DM, Jass JR, Morson BC, et al. Observer study of the grading of dysplasia in ulcerative colitis: comparison with clinical outcome. *Hum Pathol* 1989;20:1008–14.

37. Connell WR, Lennard-Jones JE, Williams CB, et al. Factors affecting the outcome of endoscopic surveillance for cancer in ulcerative colitis. *Gastroenterology* 1994;107:934–44.

38. Riddell RH. Grading of dysplasia. *Eur J Cancer* 1995;31A:1169–70.

39. Ullman T, Croog V, Harpaz N, et al. Progression of flat low-grade dysplasia to advanced neoplasia in patients with ulcerative colitis. *Gastroenterology* 2003;125:1311–19.

40. Lennard-Jones JE, Melville DM, Morson BC, et al. Precancer and cancer in extensive ulcerative colitis: findings among 401 patients over 22 years. *Gut* 1990;31:800–6.

41. Ullman TA, Loftus EV Jr, Kakar S, et al. The fate of low grade dysplasia in ulcerative colitis. *Am J Gastroenterol* 2002;97:922–7.

42. Befrits R, Ljung T, Jaramillo E, et al. Low-grade dysplasia in extensive, long-standing inflammatory bowel disease: a follow-up study. *Dis Colon Rectum* 2002;45:615–20.

43. Lim DH, Dixon MF, Vail A, et al. Ten year follow up of ulcerative colitis patients with and without low grade dysplasia. *Gut* 2003;52:1127–32.

44. Woolrich AJ, DaSilva MD, Korelitz BI. Surveillance in the routine management of ulcerative colitis: the predictive value of low-grade dysplasia. *Gastroenterology* 1992;103:431–8.

45. Karlen P, Kornfeld D, Brostrom O, et al. Is colonoscopic surveillance reducing colorectal cancer mortality in ulcerative colitis? A population based case control study. *Gut* 1998;42:711–14.

46. Griffiths AM, Sherman PM. Colonoscopic surveillance for cancer in ulcerative colitis: a critical review. *J Pediatr Gastroenterol Nutr* 1997;24:202–10.

47. Itzkowitz SH. Cancer prevention in patients with inflammatory bowel disease. *Gastroenterol Clin North Am* 2002;31:1133–44.

48. Friedman S, Rubin PH, Bodian C, et al. Screening and surveillance colonoscopy in chronic Crohn's colitis. *Gastroenterology* 2001;120:820–6.

49. Gumaste V, Sachar DB, Greenstein AJ. Benign and malignant colorectal strictures in ulcerative colitis. *Gut* 1992;33:938–41.

50. Lashner BA, Heidenreich PA, Su GL, et al. Effect of folate supplementation on the incidence of dysplasia and cancer in chronic ulcerative colitis. A case-control study. *Gastroenterology* 1989;97:255–9.

51. Lashner BA, Provencher KS, Seidner DL, et al. The effect of folic acid supplementation on the risk for cancer or dysplasia in ulcerative colitis. *Gastroenterology* 1997;112:29–32.

52. Pinczowski D, Ekbom A, Baron J, et al. Risk factors for colorectal cancer in patients with ulcerative colitis: a case-control study. *Gastroenterology* 1994;107:117–20.

53. Bansal P, Sonnenberg A. Risk factors of colorectal cancer in inflammatory bowel disease. *Am J Gastroenterol* 1996;91:44–8.

54. Bernstein CN, Blanchard JF, Metge C, et al. Does the use of 5-aminosalicylates in inflammatory bowel disease prevent the development of colorectal cancer? *Am J Gastroenterol* 2003;98:2784–8.

55. Tung BY, Emond MJ, Haggitt RC, et al. Ursodiol use is associated with lower prevalence of colonic neoplasia in patients with ulcerative colitis and primary sclerosing cholangitis. *Ann Intern Med* 2001;134:89–95.

56. Freudenheim J, Graham S, Marshall J, et al. Folate intake and carcinogenesis of the colon and rectum. *Int J Epidemiol* 1991;20:368–74.

57. Giovannucci E, Stampfer MJ, Colditz GA, et al. Folate, methionine, and alcohol intake and risk of colorectal adenoma. *J Natl Cancer Inst* 1993;85:875–84.

58. Pardi DS, Loftus EV Jr, Kremers WK, et al. Ursodeoxycholic acid as a chemopreventive agent in patients with ulcerative colitis and primary sclerosing cholangitis. *Gastroenterology* 2003;124:889–93.

59. Solem CA, Harmsen WS, Zinsmeister AR, et al. Small intestinal adenocarcinoma in Crohn's disease: a case-control study. *Inflamm Bowel Dis* 2004;10:32–5.

60. Connell WR, Sheffield JP, Kamm MA, et al. Lower gastrointestinal malignancy in Crohn's disease. *Gut* 1994;35:347–52.

61. Gullberg K, Stahlberg D, Liljeqvist L, et al. Neoplastic transformation of the pelvic pouch mucosa in patients with ulcerative colitis. *Gastroenterology* 1997;112:1487–92.

62. Thompson-Fawcett MW, Marcus V, Redston M, et al. Risk of dysplasia in long-term ileal pouches and pouches with chronic pouchitis. *Gastroenterology* 2001;121:275–81.
63. O'Riordain MG, Fazio VW, Lavery IC, et al. Incidence and natural history of dysplasia of the anal transitional zone after ileal pouch-anal anastomosis: results of a five-year to ten-year follow-up. *Dis Colon Rectum* 2000;43:1660–5.
64. Mir-Madjlessi SH, Farmer RG, Easley KA, et al. Colorectal and extracolonic malignancy in ulcerative colitis. *Cancer* 1986;58:1569–74.
65. Mellemkjaer L, Olsen JH, Frisch M, et al. Cancer in patients with ulcerative colitis. *Int J Cancer* 1995;60:330–3.
66. Karlen P, Lofberg R, Brostrom O, et al. Increased risk of cancer in ulcerative colitis: a population-based cohort study. *Am J Gastroenterol* 1999;94:1047–52.
67. Ekbom A, Helmick C, Zack M, et al. Extracolonic malignancies in inflammatory bowel disease. *Cancer* 1991;67:2015–19.
68. Greenstein AJ, Gennuso R, Sachar DB, et al. Extraintestinal cancers in inflammatory bowel disease. *Cancer* 1985;56:2914–21.
69. Caspi O, Polliack A, Klar R, et al. The association of inflammatory bowel disease and leukemia – coincidence or not? *Leuk Lymphoma* 1995;17:255–62.
70. Greenstein AJ, Mullin GE, Strauchen JA, et al. Lymphoma in inflammatory bowel disease. *Cancer* 1992;69:1119–23.
71. Persson PG, Karlen P, Bernell O, et al. Crohn's disease and cancer: a population-based cohort study. *Gastroenterology* 1994;107:1675–9.
72. Korelitz BI, Mirsky FJ, Fleisher MR, et al. Malignant neoplasms subsequent to treatment of inflammatory bowel disease with 6-mercaptopurine. *Am J Gastroenterol* 1999;94:3248–53.
73. Connell WR, Kamm MA, Dickson M, et al. Long-term neoplasia risk after azathioprine treatment in inflammatory bowel disease. *Lancet* 1994;343:1249–52.
74. Kiesslich R, Fritsch J, Holtmann M, et al. Methylene blue-aided chromoendoscopy for the detection of intraepithelial neoplasia and colon cancer in ulcerative colitis. *Gastroenterology* 2003;124:880–8.
75. Brentnall TA. Molecular underpinnings of cancer in ulcerative colitis. *Curr Opin Gastroenterol* 2003;19:64–8.
76. Ahlquist DA, Skoletsky JE, Boynton KA, et al. Colorectal cancer screening by detection of altered human DNA in stool: feasibility of a multitarget assay panel. *Gastroenterology* 2000;119:1219–27.
77. Tagore KS, Lawson MJ, Yucaitis JA, et al. Sensitivity and specificity of a stool DNA multitarget assay panel for the detection of advanced colorectal neoplasia. *Clin Colorectal Cancer* 2003;3:47–53.

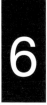

Osteoporosis: do all IBD patients need a bone density measurement?

Charles N Bernstein

Introduction

Over the past 15 years, the search for a link between osteoporosis and inflammatory bowel disease (IBD) has become a "growth industry". Several studies from tertiary referral centers have reported high rates of osteopenia and osteoporosis in IBD patients, as defined by bone density measurements. Bone density measurements are mostly performed with dual-energy x-ray absorptiometry (DXA), which is relatively inexpensive and widely accessible, although computerized tomography and ultrasound can also be used. The utility of DXA in predicting fractures has been demonstrated in postmenopausal women, older males, and corticosteroid-treated patients [1,2].

Gastroenterologists have been relatively quick to adopt the use of DXA in IBD patients. They have assumed that these measurements can predict fractures in IBD patients, as they do in postmenopausal females, even though IBD patients are often younger and the osteoporosis in IBD may have a different pathogenesis to that of the postmenopausal state. This chapter reviews the pathogenesis of osteoporosis in IBD, the prevalence of osteoporosis as assessed by DXA, and the prevalence of bone fractures in IBD. Recommendations are presented for DXA scanning in IBD patients.

Pathogenesis

Our understanding of the pathophysiology of normal bone homeostasis, the pathogenesis of osteoporosis, and the integration of osteoporosis with the immune response has been greatly advanced by the discovery of a receptor–ligand pathway identified on osteoblast and osteoclast precursors. Osteoblasts express a cell-surface ligand called RANKL (receptor activator of nuclear factor [NF]-κB ligand), which is a member of the tumor necrosis factor family. RANKL can bind either to osteoclast precursors (RANK: receptor activator of NF-κB) or to an osteoblast-derived soluble decoy receptor known as osteoprotegerin (OPG) (see **Figure 1**) [3].

This receptor–ligand interaction modulates osteoclastogenesis and, through this, the tendency for osteoporosis; alternatively, by inhibiting osteoclastogenesis and enhancing osteoblast function, this interaction can work against the development of osteoporosis. Agents that enhance RANKL production are associated with osteoporosis, whereas agents that enhance OPG production reduce osteoporosis [4]. For example, corticosteroids enhance RANKL and inhibit OPG.

In states associated with osteoporosis, patients might be expected to have higher levels of RANKL and lower levels of OPG. However, recent data have found nontraumatic fractures to be significantly associated with lower circulating RANKL levels, with the highest tertile of serum RANKL having the lowest risk of fracture [5]. In another recent report, serum OPG levels were significantly higher in patients with Crohn's disease (CD) than in those with ulcerative colitis (UC) or in population-based healthy controls [6]. Hence, rather than having a direct stimulatory (or inhibitory) effect on bone cell function, circulating levels of RANKL and OPG may be a response to processes occurring at the cellular level. For instance, lower circulating RANKL levels may be a response to reduced bone mass; and elevated circulating OPG in CD patients may be

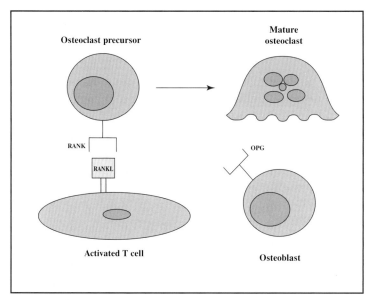

Figure 1. The RANKL–RANK–OPG receptor–ligand pathway.

a response to reduced bone mass in CD. Alternatively, altered RANKL (or OPG) levels in CD patients may reflect the circulating lymphocyte status or even colonic dendritic cell release.

Studies in animal models

RANKL is a regulator of T cell–dendritic cell interaction in the immune system, and is a crucial factor in early lymphocyte development and lymph node organogenesis [7]. *Rankl*-deficient mice lack all lymph nodes [8].

The interleukin (IL)-2-deficient mouse model of colitis develops both osteopenia and colitis [9]. In a recent report, IL-2-deficient mice had elevated bone marrow mononuclear cell expression of RANKL and OPG mRNA, and raised circulating serum RANKL and OPG (an example where OPG levels were elevated in the presence of definite osteopenia) compared with control littermates. Osteopenia could be induced in T-cell-deficient mice by the adoptive transfer of T cells from IL-2-deficient mice [9]. This suggests that activated T cells are critical in mediating osteopenia. Exogenous OPG administration reversed both osteopenia and colitis.

This study also showed that dendritic cells are the main colon cells that respond to OPG. Overall, these data underscore the importance of OPG in osteopenia and colitis in IL-2-deficient mice, and the importance of activated T cells in mediating these conditions. These data may provide the link between an inflammatory condition such as CD and the development of osteoporosis. This connection may be via the RANK–RANKL–OPG receptor–ligand pathway, and may occur between lymphopoietic cells, including T cells and dendritic cells, as well as osteoclasts and osteoblasts.

Corticosteroids and fracture risk

Many studies have examined the correlation between disease activity, disease location, past surgeries, corticosteroid use, and changes in bone density, but no clear consensus has emerged from the data [10]. While corticosteroids can affect RANKL and OPG, less than 50% of fractures in CD patients and less than 20% of fractures in UC patients are associated with corticosteroid use [11]. A small, population-based study of fractures from Olmsted County, USA, did not find an association between corticosteroid use and fractures in CD patients [12].

Recently, a population-based case-control study from Manitoba, Canada, assessed the association between corticosteroid use and fractures [13]. No association was evident for UC. However, approximately half of the CD patients who fractured were using corticosteroids; this was significantly more than the matched CD subjects who had not fractured. This study could not distinguish the effect of corticosteroid use from the effect of active inflammatory disease (this has always been a problem with assessing corticosteroid use in IBD: is it the drugs or the active inflammation the drugs are treating that is associated with the lower bone mass?). However, this study does suggest that patients with sufficiently active disease to warrant corticosteroids have an increased risk for fracture.

It is also clear from the above studies that corticosteroids are neither necessary for fracturing in IBD, nor sufficient in themselves to cause a fracture, since many corticosteroid users do not fracture [13]. While the medical literature does associate corticosteroids with fracturing, the data have mostly been drawn from the rheumatic disease literature, which represents, on average, an older population than that of IBD patients.

Can IBD patients be stratified for fracture risk?

The literature suggests that 15% of IBD patients have bone density in the osteoporotic range, while approximately 50% have bone density in the osteopenic range [10]. The osteopenic range (T score between –1 and –2.5; see **Table 1**) is associated with a heightened fracture risk in postmenopausal females and corticosteroid users; however, the osteopenic range is also part of the normal distribution among healthy adults. Hence, while many patients with IBD will have DXA scans that suggest bone density in the range of osteopenia, they may actually not be at any greater risk than at least 20% of the healthy population. Furthermore, these DXA studies have mostly been from tertiary referral centers and, therefore, represent a skewed population.

These data, together with expert recommendations for pursuing an aggressive DXA scanning and therapeutic intervention strategy [14–17], have led practicing gastroenterologists to consider DXA scanning for all IBD patients, and aggressive bisphosphonate use in all corticosteroid users and many noncorticosteroid users who have any suggestion of lower bone density (including osteopenia). The main flaw in this strategy is that the fracture data for IBD do not justify this approach.

T score	Interpretation
Above –1	Normal
–1 to –2.5	Osteopenia
Below –2.5	Osteoporosis

Table 1. The T score: the number of standard deviations above or below the average peak young-adult bone mineral density.

Studies of fracture risk

There have been four population-based studies of fracture risk in IBD [11,12,18,19]. The first to be published was from Manitoba [18]. The incidence of fracture was approximately 1/100 patient-years in approximately 40,000 patient-years of risk. Compared with the age- and gender-matched non-IBD general population, the incidence rate ratio in this study was 1.41 (95% confidence interval 1.27–1.56). This suggests a statistically significant, but not very large, increased risk; the incidence rate indicates that fractures are not actually that common. The data from this study showed that fractures are most common among IBD patients over the age of 60 years, and that both CD and UC patients are similarly affected.

Population-based studies from the UK and Denmark have shown comparably low, but statistically significant, increased risks of fracture in IBD patients compared with non-IBD populations – this increase is in the order of 1.2-fold [11,19]. Both of these studies showed a correlation between increasing age and increasing fracture risk. Finally, a study from Olmsted County did not show an overall increased fracture risk among CD patients, but did show a trend towards an increased risk of osteoporosis-associated fractures with increasing age [12].

A further piece of evidence supporting the notion that fractures and osteoporosis are not major issues for most young IBD patients was reported in another Manitoba study. Using the University of Manitoba IBD Research Registry (a Registry of approximately half of Manitoba's IBD population, and of subjects who allow future contacts for other studies), females under the age of 45 years who were diagnosed with IBD prior to the age of 20 years were asked to participate in the study (because their IBD was diagnosed at a young age, these women are considered to be a high-risk cohort) [20]. Once premenopausal status was confirmed, the subjects completed questionnaires and underwent DXA scanning. Surprisingly, only 3% had bone density in the osteoporotic range and, on average, the bone densities of these women were similar to those of age-matched controls. Hence, even among this supposedly high-risk cohort, their bone densities as premenopausal adults were mostly normal.

Risk stratification

While smoking, hypogonadism, lack of exercise, family history of osteoporosis, and personal past fracture history are key components of fracture risk (as they are in the non-IBD population), it seems that IBD poses an additional risk factor. However, it is uncertain how to weight this risk factor juxtaposed to any of the other known risk factors. It is clear that elderly IBD patients have the highest risk among the IBD population, so clinicians should remember to address the bone status of this IBD cohort in particular.

Corticosteroid-using CD patients, regardless of age, are also at increased risk for osteoporosis, either from their active disease or from the drug itself; however, it is unclear when the risk really begins. Although corticosteroids can be associated with an early fracture risk, withdrawal of corticosteroids is associated with a rapid diminution of the fracture risk [21]. Therefore, it may be unnecessary to put a young person on a bisphosphonate or order a DXA scan at the time of initiating corticosteroids, considering that they may be off corticosteroids in the very near future and that their bone mass will rebound. It remains unclear which aspect of corticosteroid dosing poses the greatest risk to bones: is it the first dose of prednisone administered, or after corticosteroids have been administered for some length of time? A recent study suggests that the daily dose is a greater predictor of fracture risk than the cumulative dose [22].

Figure 2 presents an approach to DXA scanning in IBD. An important feature of this paradigm is that all patients with past low-impact vertebral fractures should be treated as if they have osteoporosis, regardless of their bone density. It is known that only about one third of postmenopausal fractures occur in patients with DXA results in the osteoporotic range, so a normal DXA scan does not provide full reassurance about fracture risk [23]. It has also been shown that only 38% of an IBD population with fractures had spine bone mineral density in the osteoporotic range [24]. Since a past vertebral fracture is a risk factor for future fracture, it might be worth pursuing spine x-rays to assess for silent vertebral fractures. Although this may seem to be a simple approach, it is not without problems, since assessing spine x-rays for fracture is not foolproof [25]; vertebral fractures are often under-reported on plain x-rays.

In summary, the major risk factors for fracture among IBD patients are age and chronically active corticosteroid-requiring disease (somewhat arbitrarily set at 3 months of corticosteroid use). These should dictate the majority of DXA scanning in IBD. However, the usual risk factors for osteoporosis and fractures are also relevant to IBD patients and may dictate interventions.

Treatment of osteoporosis in IBD

Nutritional supplements

Patients with IBD should maintain an adequate calcium intake (1,000 mg/day elemental calcium for individuals <50 years old; 1,500 mg/day for those >50 years old) and vitamin D intake (400–800 IU/day). Typically, IBD patients have a suboptimal intake of these bone-modifying nutrients [26,27] and – in view of the potential for reduced intake because of anorexia, malabsorption, or simply intolerance to foods high in calcium

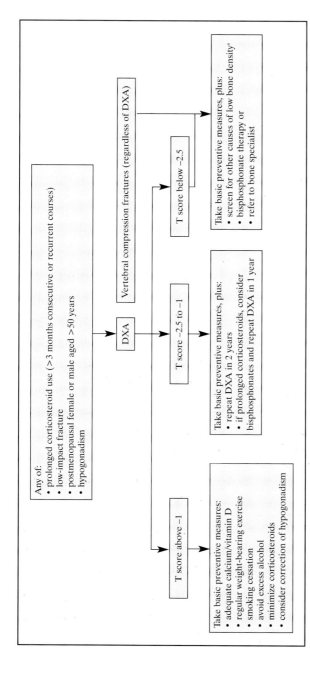

Figure 2. An approach to DXA (dual-energy x-ray absorptiometry) scanning in inflammatory bowel disease patients. [a]Complete blood count, serum calcium, alkaline phosphatase, creatinine, 25-OH-vitamin D, protein electrophoresis, testosterone (males). Adapted with permission from the American Gastroenterological Association (Bernstein CN, Leslie WD, Leboff MS. AGA technical review on osteoporosis in gastrointestinal diseases. *Gastroenterology* 2003;124:795–841).

content – it may be that IBD patients should be uniformly supplemented with calcium and vitamin D. However, since many patients with IBD are in clinical remission for prolonged periods and eat robust diets, supplementation is unnecessary in all patients. In addition, it has recently been shown that calcium and vitamin D intake does not correlate with bone mineral density [26].

My standard approach is to recommend these supplements to IBD patients when it is determined that they have low bone density, they are initiated on corticosteroids, they have known hypogonadism or are postmenopausal, or they have sustained a fracture. In northern climates, such as most of Canada, the northern US, and northern Europe, vitamin D supplementation may be of enhanced importance since direct contact with sunlight is limited during fall and the winter months. It is important to ensure adequate calcium and vitamin D intake, as they may have long-term bone effects.

Bisphosphonates

Bisphosphonates are an important adjunctive treatment in those with low bone density who are thought to be at particularly high risk for fracture. Their utility is not in question in postmenopausal and corticosteroid-associated osteoporosis. However, the endpoint for bisphosphonate use has yet to be clarified in IBD patients. If initiated in a corticosteroid-using patient, should bisphosphonates be taken only during corticosteroid dosing? (This approach is problematic, as some have shown only minimal changes in bone density over time during corticosteroid dosing [10]; also, some patients may use repeated short courses of corticosteroids.) Should bisphosphonates be continued until the patient's disease is in remission? Should they be continued indefinitely? How safe is their use in women of child-bearing age, and what should be done if the patient becomes pregnant while on bisphosphonates? These questions regarding the endpoint of bisphosphonate use must be weighed against an absence of proof that bisphosphonates (which are generally poorly absorbed in a normal subject) will prevent fractures in younger patients with IBD.

Referral

There are several complex issues at play in those IBD patients with an increased risk for fracture. In general, fracture prevention in high-risk IBD patients might be best handled by a bone specialist. For postmenopausal women, issues regarding hormone supplementation have become increasingly complex with the publication of data underscoring the potentially high risk of this approach [28]. In men, recent evidence has suggested that serum estrogen may be more important than androgens in regulating bone mass [29,30]. Hence, sex hormone assessment in relation to bone mass (even in males) may be more complex than simply measuring serum testosterone. Another reason for considering referral to a bone specialist is that new therapies are evolving for patients who are intolerant to bisphosphonates or even for those who are using these agents, but require additional therapy [10]. The bone specialist will be best positioned to fully explore these options with the patient.

Primary prevention advice can be easily undertaken by the gastroenterologist managing IBD patients. This includes dietary advice, simple supplementation, advice against smoking, assessment of sex hormone status, encouraging exercise, treating active inflammation, and limiting corticosteroids. However, pharmacologic prevention and intervention might be best managed by a bone specialist.

Clinical vignettes

Case 1

A 24-year-old woman with newly diagnosed ileal CD has been treated with prednisone 40 mg/day for the past 2 months. She does not smoke and has regular menses. She has never had a low-impact fracture.

Prescribe calcium and vitamin D supplementation?
Yes. Supplementation with 1,000 mg/day of calcium and 800 IU/day of vitamin D should be encouraged.

Perform DXA?
No.

Prescribe bisphosphonates?
No. This woman is at low risk for sustaining a fracture in the near future. She may be off corticosteroids within 3 months.

After 3 months off prednisone the woman returns feeling well. It is elected to maintain her on mesalamine 4 g/day. She became tired of taking the calcium and vitamin D supplements and stopped 3 weeks prior to the appointment.

Restart calcium and vitamin D supplementation?
No, not if her diet is replete with these. If it is not then she will need supplements.

Perform DXA?
No.

Prescribe bisphosphonates?
No.

Case 2

A 32-year-old male with a 20-year history of CD is on azathioprine 150 mg/day. He has had recurrent courses of prednisone, the last of which was 1 year prior to this appointment. He has had three small bowel resections and his rectum and sigmoid have been removed, leaving him with an end-descending colostomy. Past courses of methotrexate and infliximab have been unsuccessful. He has a percutaneous gastrostomy feeding tube that he uses intermittently when his tolerance for oral intake is diminished. He is mostly sedentary. His serum testosterone level is normal.

Prescribe calcium and vitamin D supplementation?
Yes (indefinite use).

Perform DXA?
Yes. He has had chronic active disease and considerable cumulative corticosteroids, he is sedentary, and his nutrition is questionable at times.

Prescribe bisphosphonates?
No.

His DXA scan result reveals a T score of +2.2 at the spine and +2.4 at the hip. Despite this normal bone density, he still carries some risk factors for fracture; however, it is not possible to quantify the risk. Nonetheless, there is no indication for bisphosphonates.

Case 3

A 53-year-old woman with CD comes in for an annual review. She was diagnosed with CD 12 years ago. She used prednisone for 4 months after her initial diagnosis, but has not used it since. She feels very well on no medication. She had an ileal resection 2 years ago when she presented with an acute obstruction. Her last menstrual period was 5 years ago. She has not had a low-impact fracture. She drinks four glasses of milk a day.

Prescribe calcium and vitamin D supplementation?
Unlikely to be necessary with her milk intake, but a more complete dietary history should be taken to substantiate that she takes in 1,500 mg/day of calcium and 800 IU/day of vitamin D.

Perform DXA?
Yes. She is postmenopausal and her CD presents some risk for fracture.

Prescribe bisphosphonates?
Wait until DXA results are available.

Her DXA scan reveals a T score of –2.6 at the hip and –1.4 at the spine. One study has suggested an increased risk for fracture with more active disease [11], but other studies have not correlated fracture with disease activity. Therefore, although this patient is in disease remission, she is not necessarily protected from having a fracture risk from CD. Her hip T score is in the osteoporosis range. Because she is a postmenopausal female, one approach to preventing hip fracture would be to use estrogen replacement therapy, particularly if she has postmenopausal symptoms. Another therapeutic intervention to consider would be bisphosphonates. Hence, she should be referred to a bone specialist for advice on therapy.

Case 4

A 57-year-old woman who has had UC for 22 years presents with the first flare of her colitis for 4 years. She is usually maintained on sulfasalazine 4 g/day, but she stopped her sulfasalazine 3 months ago. One year ago she underwent a DXA scan, which revealed a T score of –1.2 at the hip and –1.3 at the spine. She is now treated with prednisone 40 mg/day. She had a hysterectomy 9 years ago. She exercises regularly and has not had a low-impact fracture. She has a full diet, including raw vegetables, but eats few dairy products.

Prescribe calcium and vitamin D supplementation?
Yes.

Perform DXA?
No.

Prescribe bisphosphonates?
No.

She requires calcium and vitamin D supplementation since she is postmenopausal and starting corticosteroids, and may not be ingesting adequate calcium and vitamin D. Her DXA results from 1 year ago were not even in the osteopenic range. If she can easily come off prednisone and resume her sulfasalazine maintenance then it would be reasonable to retake her DXA measurements in 1 year (2–3 years after her last test). She does not require bisphosphonates if she is able to withdraw from prednisone easily; however, if it is projected that she will require a prolonged course of corticosteroids (for longer than 3 months) then bisphosphonates might be indicated.

References

1. Cummings SR, Black DM, Nevitt MC, et al. Bone density at various sites for prediction of hip fractures. The Study of Osteoporotic Fractures Research Group. *Lancet* 1993;341:72–5.
2. Van Staa TP, Laan RF, Barton IP, et al. Bone density threshold and other predictors of vertebral fracture in patients receiving oral glucocorticoid therapy. *Arthritis Rheum* 2003;48:3224–9.
3. Khosla S. Minireview: the OPG/RANKL/RANK system. *Endocrinology* 2001;142:5050–5.
4. Kong YY, Penninger JM. Molecular control of bone remodeling and osteoporosis. *Exp Gerontol* 2000;35:947–56.
5. Schett G, Kiechl S, Redlich K, et al. Soluble RANKL and risk of nontraumatic fracture. *JAMA* 2004;291:1108–13.
6. Bernstein CN, Sargent M, Leslie WD. Serum osteoprotegerin is increased in Crohn's disease: A population-based case control study. *Gastroenterology* 2004;126:A469 (Abstr.).
7. Kong YY, Boyle WJ, Penninger JM. Osteoprotegerin ligand: a common link between osteoclastogenesis, lymph node formation and lymphocyte development. *Immunol Cell Biol* 1999;77:188–93.
8. Kong YY, Feige U, Sarosi I, et al. Activated T cells regulate bone loss and joint destruction in adjuvant arthritis through osteoprotegerin ligand. *Nature* 1999;402:304–9.
9. Ashcroft AJ, Cruickshank SM, Croucher PI, et al. Colonic dendritic cells, intestinal inflammation, and T cell-mediated bone destruction are modulated by recombinant osteoprotegerin. *Immunity* 2003;19:849–61.
10. Bernstein CN, Leslie WD, Leboff MS. AGA technical review on osteoporosis in gastrointestinal diseases. *Gastroenterology* 2003;124:795–841.
11. van Staa TP, Cooper C, Brusse LS, et al. Inflammatory bowel disease and the risk of fracture. *Gastroenterology* 2003;125:1591–7.
12. Loftus EV Jr, Crowson CS, Sandborn WJ, et al. Long-term fracture risk in patients with Crohn's disease: a population-based study in Olmsted County, Minnesota. *Gastroenterology* 2002;123:468–75.
13. Bernstein CN, Blanchard JF, Metge C, et al. The association between corticosteroid use and development of fractures among IBD patients in a population-based database. *Am J Gastroenterol* 2003;98:1797–801.
14. Buchman AL. Bones and Crohn's: problems and solutions. *Inflamm Bowel Dis* 1999;5:212–27.
15. Compston JE. Review article: osteoporosis, corticosteroids and inflammatory bowel disease. *Aliment Pharmacol Ther* 1995;9:237–50.
16. De Vos M, De Keyser F, Mielants H, et al. Review article: bone and joint diseases in inflammatory bowel disease. *Aliment Pharmacol Ther* 1998;12:397–404.
17. Valentine JF, Sninsky CA. Prevention and treatment of osteoporosis in patients with inflammatory bowel disease. *Am J Gastroenterol* 1999;94:878–83.
18. Bernstein CN, Blanchard JF, Leslie WD, et al. The incidence of fracture among patients with inflammatory bowel disease. A population-based cohort study. *Ann Intern Med* 2000;133:795–9.
19. Vestergaard P, Mosekilde L. Fracture risk in patients with celiac disease, Crohn's disease, and ulcerative colitis: a nationwide follow-up study of 16,416 patients in Denmark. *Am J Epidemiol* 2002;156:1–10.
20. Bernstein CN, Leslie WD, Taback S. Bone density in a population-based cohort of premenopausal adult women with early onset inflammatory bowel disease. *Am J Gastroenterol* 2003;98:1094–100.

21. van Staa TP, Leufkens HG, Cooper C. The epidemiology of corticosteroid-induced osteoporosis: a meta-analysis. *Osteoporos Int* 2002;13:777–87.
22. van Staa TP, Laan RF, Barton IP, et al. Bone density threshold and other predictors of vertebral fracture in patients receiving oral glucocorticoid therapy. *Arthritis Rheum* 2003;48:3224–9.
23. Espallargues M, Sampietro-Colom L, Estrada MD, et al. Identifying bone-mass-related risk factors for fracture to guide bone densitometry measurements: a systematic review of the literature. *Osteoporos Int* 2001;12:811–22.
24. Klaus J, Armbrecht G, Steinkamp M, et al. High prevalence of osteoporotic vertebral fractures in patients with Crohn's disease. *Gut* 2002;51:654–8.
25. Gehlbach SH, Bigelow C, Heimisdottir M, et al. Recognition of vertebral fracture in a clinical setting. *Osteoporos Int* 2000;11:577–82.
26. Bernstein CN, Bector S, Leslie WD. Lack of relationship of calcium and vitamin D intake to bone mineral density in premenopausal women with inflammatory bowel disease. *Am J Gastroenterol* 2003;98:2468–73.
27. Bernstein CN, Seeger LL, Anton PA, et al. A randomized, placebo-controlled trial of calcium supplementation for decreased bone density in corticosteroid-using patients with inflammatory bowel disease: a pilot study. *Aliment Pharmacol Ther* 1996;10:777–86.
28. Rossouw JE, Anderson GL, Prentice RL, et al. Risks and benefits of estrogen plus progestin in healthy postmenopausal women: principal results from the Women's Health Initiative randomized controlled trial. *JAMA* 2002;288:321–33.
29. Gennari L, Merlotti D, Martini G, et al. Longitudinal association between sex hormone levels, bone loss, and bone turnover in elderly men. *J Clin Endocrinol Metab* 2003;88:5327–33.
30. Khosla S, Melton LJ 3rd, Riggs BL. Clinical review 144: estrogen and the male skeleton. *J Clin Endocrinol Metab* 2002;87:1443–50.

Abbreviations

5-ASA	5-aminosalicylate
ASCA	anti-*Saccharomyces cerevisiae* antibody
CARD	caspase recruitment domain
CD	Crohn's disease
CDAI	Crohn's disease activity index
CI	confidence interval
CRC	colorectal cancer
DALM	dysplasia-associated lesion or mass
DXA	dual-energy x-ray absorptiometry
GI	gastrointestinal
HGD	high-grade dysplasia
HLA	human leukocyte antigen
IAA	ileoanal anastomosis
IBD	inflammatory bowel disease
Ig	immunoglobulin
IL	interleukin
IPAA	ileal pouch-anal anastomosis
IRA	ileorectal anastomosis
LGD	low-grade dysplasia
MDP	muramyl dipeptide
mdr	multidrug resistance gene
mRNA	messenger RNA
NF	nuclear factor
NOD	nucleotide-binding oligomerization domain
NSAIDs	nonsteroidal anti-inflammatory drugs
OmpC	outer membrane porin protein C
OPG	osteoprotegerin

OVA	ovalbumin
pANCA	perinuclear anti-neutrophil cytoplasmic antibody
PCR	polymerase chain reaction
PEG	percutaneous endoscopic gastrostomy
PSC	primary sclerosing cholangitis
RANK	receptor activator of nuclear factor-κB
RANKL	receptor activator of nuclear factor-κB ligand
SCID	severe combined immunodeficiency
SIR	standardized incidence ratio
TAP	transporter associated with antigen processing
TCR	T-cell receptor
Th	T-helper cell
TNF	tumor necrosis factor
TPN	total parenteral nutrition
Treg	regulatory T cell
UC	ulcerative colitis

Index

Page numbers in **bold** refer to figures.
Page numbers in *italics* refer to tables.